Dietary Reference Intakes Research Synthesis Workshop Summary

Carol West Suitor and Linda D. Meyers, *Rapporteurs*

Food and Nutrition Board

INSTITUTE OF MEDICINE
OF THE NATIONAL ACADEMIES

THE NATIONAL ACADEMIES PRESS
Washington, D.C.
www.nap.edu

THE NATIONAL ACADEMIES PRESS 500 Fifth Street, N.W. Washington, DC 20001

NOTICE: The project that is the subject of this report was approved by the Governing Board of the National Research Council, whose members are drawn from the councils of the National Academy of Sciences, the National Academy of Engineering, and the Institute of Medicine. The members of the planning committee responsible for the workshop were chosen for their special competences and with regard for appropriate balance.

The study was supported by Contract No. HHSP23320042509XI, Task Order No. 05 between the National Academy of Sciences and the United States Department of Health and Human Services; by Grant No. 59-0790-5-183 from the United States Department of Agriculture; by Contract No. 4500096095 with Health Canada; and by a grant from the Candian Institues of Health Research (through Simon Frasier University). Any opinions, findings, conclusions, or recommendations expressed in this publication are those of the authors and do not necessarily reflect the views of the organizations or agencies that provided support for the project.

International Standard Book Number-10: 0-309-10322-3
International Standard Book Number-13: 978-0-309-10322-0

Additional copies of this report are available from the National Academies Press, 500 Fifth Street, N.W., Box 285, Washington, DC 20055. Call (800) 624-6242 or (202) 334-3313 (in the Washington metropolitan area), Internet, http://www.nap.edu.

For more information about the Institute of Medicine, visit the IOM home page at: **www.iom.edu.**

Printed in the United States of America.

The serpent has been a symbol of long life, healing, and knowledge among almost all cultures and religions since the beginning of recorded history. The serpent adopted as a logotype by the Institute of Medicine is a relief carving from ancient Greece, now held by the Staatliche Museen in Berlin.

"Knowing is not enough; we must apply.
Willing is not enough; we must do."
—Goethe

INSTITUTE OF MEDICINE
OF THE NATIONAL ACADEMIES

Advising the Nation. Improving Health.

THE NATIONAL ACADEMIES

Advisers to the Nation on Science, Engineering, and Medicine

The **National Academy of Sciences** is a private, nonprofit, self-perpetuating society of distinguished scholars engaged in scientific and engineering research, dedicated to the furtherance of science and technology and to their use for the general welfare. Upon the authority of the charter granted to it by the Congress in 1863, the Academy has a mandate that requires it to advise the federal government on scientific and technical matters Dr. Ralph J. Cicerone is president of the National Academy of Sciences.

The **National Academy of Engineering** was established in 1964, under the charter of the National Academy of Sciences, as a parallel organization of outstanding engineers. It is autonomous in its administration and in the selection of its members, sharing with the National Academy of Sciences the responsibility for advising the federal government. The National Academy of Engineering also sponsors engineering programs aimed at meeting national needs, encourages education and research, and recognizes the superior achievements of engineers. Dr. Wm. A. Wulf is president of the National Academy of Engineering.

The **Institute of Medicine** was established in 1970 by the National Academy of Sciences to secure the services of eminent members of appropriate professions in the examination of policy matters pertaining to the health of the public. The Institute acts under the responsibility given to the National Academy of Sciences by its congressional charter to be an adviser to the federal government and, upon its own initiative, to identify issues of medical care, research, and education. Dr. Harvey V. Fineberg is president of the Institute of Medicine.

The **National Research Council** was organized by the National Academy of Sciences in 1916 to associate the broad community of science and technology with the Academy's purposes of furthering knowledge and advising the federal government. Functioning in accordance with general policies determined by the Academy, the Council has become the principal operating agency of both the National Academy of Sciences and the National Academy of Engineering in providing services to the government, the public, and the scientific and engineering communities. The Council is administered jointly by both Academies and the Institute of Medicine. Dr. Ralph J. Cicerone and Dr. Wm. A. Wulf are chair and vice chair, respectively, of the National Research Council.

www.national-academies.org

PLANNING COMMITTEE ON DIETARY REFERENCE INTAKES RESEARCH SYNTHESIS

JOHN W. SUTTIE *(Chair)*, Department of Biochemistry, University of Wisconsin, Madison
JOHN W. ERDMAN, JR., Department of Food Science and Human Nutrition, University of Illinois at Urbana-Champaign
SUZANNE P. MURPHY, Cancer Research Center of Hawaii, University of Hawaii, Honolulu
ROBERT M. RUSSELL, Jean Mayer USDA Human Nutrition Research Center on Aging, Tufts University, Boston, MA
SUSAN WHITING, Division of Nutrition and Dietetics, College of Pharmacy and Nutrition, University of Saskatchewan, Saskatoon, Saskatchewan

Consultant Writer
CAROL WEST SUITOR, Nutrition Consultant, Northfield, Vermont,

Staff
LINDA D. MEYERS, Study Director (from July 2006)
JANICE RICE OKITA, Study Director (until July 2006)
HEATHER DEL VALLE, Senior Program Assistant and Database Manager

FOOD AND NUTRITION BOARD*

DENNIS M. BIER *(Chair)*, Children's Nutrition Research Center, Baylor College of Medicine, Houston, TX
MICHAEL P. DOYLE *(Vice Chair)*, Center for Food Safety, University of Georgia, Griffin
DIANE BIRT, Center for Research on Dietary Botanical Supplements, Iowa State University, Ames
YVONNE BRONNER, School of Public Health and Policy, Morgan State University, Baltimore, MD
SUSAN FERENC, Chemical Producers and Distributors Association, Alexandria, VA
NANCY F. KREBS, Department of Pediatrics, University of Colorado Health Sciences Center, Denver
REYNALDO MARTORELL, Hubert Department of Global Health, Rollins School of Public Health, Emory University, Atlanta, GA
J. GLENN MORRIS, JR., Department of Epidemiology and Preventive Medicine, University of Maryland School of Medicine, Baltimore
SUZANNE P. MURPHY, Cancer Research Center of Hawaii, University of Hawaii, Honolulu
JOSE M. ORDOVAS, Jean Mayer USDA Human Nutrition Research Center on Aging, Tufts University, Boston, MA
JIM E. RIVIERE, College of Veterinary Medicine, North Carolina State University, Raleigh
NICHOLAS J. SCHORK, Department of Psychiatry, Polymorphism Research Laboratory, University of California, San Diego
REBECCA J. STOLTZFUS, Division of Nutritional Sciences, Cornell University, Ithaca, NY
JOHN W. SUTTIE, Department of Biochemistry, University of Wisconsin, Madison
WALTER C. WILLETT, Department of Nutrition, Harvard School of Public Health, Boston, MA
BARRY L. ZOUMAS, Department of Agricultural Economics and Rural Sociology, Pennsylvania State University, University Park

Staff
LINDA D. MEYERS, Director
GERALDINE KENNEDO, Administrative Assistant
ANTON L. BANDY, Financial Associate

*IOM boards do not review or approve individual reports and are not asked to endorse conclusions and recommendations. The responsibility for the content of the report rests with the authoring committee and the institution.

Independent Report Reviewers

This report has been reviewed in draft form by individuals chosen for their diverse perspectives and technical expertise, in accordance with procedures approved by the National Research Council's Report Review Committee. The purpose of this independent review is to provide candid and critical comments that will assist the institution in making its published report as sound as possible and to ensure that the report meets institutional standards for objectivity, evidence, and responsiveness to the study charge. The review comments and draft manuscript remain confidential to protect the integrity of the deliberative process. We wish to thank the following individuals for their review of this report:

STEPHANIE A. ATKINSON, Department of Pediatrics, McMaster University, Hamilton, Ontario, Canada
JOHN W. ERDMAN, JR., Department of Food Science and Human Nutrition, University of Illinois at Urbana-Champaign
A. CATHARINE ROSS, Department of Nutritional Sciences, The Pennsylvania State University, University Park
JOHN W. SUTTIE, Department of Biochemistry, University of Wisconsin, Madison

Although the reviewers listed above have provided many constructive comments and suggestions, they were not asked to endorse the final draft of the report before its release. The review of this report was overseen by **MELVIN WORTH**, Scholar-in-Residence at the Institute of Medicine, who was appointed by the Institute of Medicine. He was responsible for making certain that an independent examination of this report was carried out in accordance with institutional procedures and that all review comments were carefully considered.

Contents

Overview

DIETARY REFERENCE INTAKES RESEARCH SYNTHESIS WORKSHOP

What information is available to inform the planning of a nutrition research agenda for the United States and Canada? This question provided the backdrop for the Dietary Reference Intakes Research Synthesis project undertaken by the Food and Nutrition Board of the Institute of Medicine (IOM) of the National Academies. The Dietary Reference Intakes (DRIs) are quantitative reference values for recommended intakes and tolerable upper intake levels for a range of nutrients. They are used widely by dietitians in individual counseling, by federal nutrition officials in program and policy development, and by the nutrition research and education communities in government, academia, and industry.

Between 1997 and 2005, the IOM published a series of six DRI reports covering a total of 45 nutrients, energy, and other food components. The IOM also issued two reports describing ways to apply the DRIs in assessment and planning. Together, these eight reports contain more than 450 research recommendations and thus a wealth of information pertinent to a nutrition research agenda. To make the recommendations more accessible, the Food and Nutrition Board undertook a project with two major elements: (1) the development of a searchable database of all the DRI research recommendations, and (2) the Dietary Reference Intakes Research Synthesis Workshop, held June 7–8, 2006, which was designed to provide a venue for hearing and discussing experts' perspectives on the research recommendations identified in the DRI reports. Appendix A contains the agenda for the workshop, and Appendix B lists the names and affiliations of meeting presenters and other participants, including members of the Federal DRI Research Synthesis Subcommittee, which supported the workshop and provided useful substantive input.

The project was sponsored by the U.S. and Canadian governments, specifically:

- U.S. Department of Health and Human Services
  National Institutes of Health, Division of Nutrition Research Coordination
  National Institutes of Health, Office of Dietary Supplements
  Office of Disease Prevention and Health Promotion
- U.S. Department of Agriculture, Agricultural Research Service
- Health Canada, Food Directorate, Bureau of Nutritional Sciences
- Canadian Institutes of Health Research, Institute of Nutrition, Metabolism and Diabetes

THE WORKSHOP

Two members of the workshop planning group—Drs. John W. Suttie and Susan J. Whiting—moderated the DRI Research Synthesis Workshop. After an overview and demonstration of the DRI Research Synthesis Database, panels of experts addressed DRI research recommendations related to each of the six DRI nutrient reports, the two DRI applications reports, and three cross-cutting topics: (1) setting DRIs for children, (2) Tolerable Upper Intake Levels, and (3) relevant new and underutilized research techniques. Periodically, presenters and other attendees took part in lively discussions. During the wrap-up session, moderator John Suttie and four other individuals—from U.S. and Canadian agencies, industry, and academia—provided their perspectives on the workshop.

This report is a summary of the workshop presentations and discussions. Meeting transcripts and slides used during presentations served as the basis for the summary. Topics frequently mentioned by individual participants as continuing knowledge gaps include the following:

- Requirements of children, pregnant and lactating women, and the elderly
- Individual variation of requirements caused by genetics and epigenetics, lifestyle, environment, and/or geography
- The need for biomarkers that are able to predict functional outcomes and chronic diseases

- The need to improve dietary assessments and planning methods
- Bioavailability
- Interactions among nutrients

Although many presenters and discussants expressed strong viewpoints and made research recommendations, their viewpoints and recommendations should not be viewed as workshop conclusions or recommendations. For the convenience of users of the DRI recommendations, Appendix C lists all the research recommendations made in the eight DRI reports, Appendix D provides an overview of the DRI Research Synthesis Database, Appendix E lists research progress as reported by presenters, Appendix F lists possible topics for research identified during the workshop, and Appendix G provides the meaning of abbreviations.

1

Introductory Session[1]

During the opening session of the workshop, two representatives of sponsoring agencies—Paul M. Coates from the U.S. government and Peter Fischer from the Canadian government—described the goals of the Dietary Reference Intake Research Synthesis project and its potential uses. Then John W. Erdman, Jr., described the approach and framework of the Dietary Reference Intakes (DRIs). Dr. Erdman served as a member, vice-chair, and then chair of the Standing Committee on Scientific Evaluation of Dietary Reference Intakes that oversaw the 1994–2004 DRI process.

OVERVIEW

Presenters: Paul M. Coates and Peter Fischer

Goals of the Project

The main goal for the workshop was a discussion of expert perspectives on the research needs that have been identified in eight DRI reports (see Box 1-1). Taking part in the discussion were many of those who worked on the DRI reports, including some former chairs of DRI panels, other former committee and panel members, and many other experts (see Appendix B).

---

[1]This chapter is an edited version of remarks by Drs. Coates, Fischer, and Erdman at the workshop.

BOX 1-1
Dietary Reference Intake Reports

Complete Title	**Letter Designation and Abbreviated Title**	**Year of Publication***
Dietary Reference Intakes for Calcium, Phosphorus, Magnesium, Vitamin D, and Fluoride	A Calcium and Related Nutrients Report	1997
Dietary Reference Intakes for Thiamin, Riboflavin, Niacin, Vitamin B6, Folate, Vitamin B12, Pantothenic Acid, Biotin, and Choline	B B Vitamins and Choline Report	1998
Dietary Reference Intakes for Vitamin C, Vitamin E, Selenium, and Carotenoids	C Antioxidants Report	2000
Dietary Reference Intakes for Vitamin A, Vitamin K, Arsenic, Boron, Chromium, Copper, Iodine, Iron, Manganese, Molybdenum, Nickel, Silicon, Vanadium, and Zinc	D Micronutrients Report	2001
Dietary Reference Intakes for Energy, Carbohydrate, Fiber, Fat, Fatty Acids, Cholesterol, Protein, and Amino Acids	E Macronutrients Report	2002/2005
Dietary Reference Intakes: Water, Potassium, Sodium, Chloride, and Sulfate	F Electrolytes and Water Report	2005
Dietary Reference Intakes: Applications in Dietary Assessment	G Assessment Report	2000
Dietary Reference Intakes: Applications in Dietary Planning	H Planning Report	2003

* Also refers to the year a report was released, except for Reports E and F, which were released as prepublication (uncorrected proof) copies, in 2002 and 2004, respectively.

A federal steering committee, which has both U.S. and Canadian participants, was actively involved in planning for this project. The Federal DRI Steering Committee represents a wide range of interest in the

DRIs. (See Appendix B for a listing of committee members and the agencies they represent.) Dr. Coates, a member of the steering committee and cochairperson of its research synthesis subcommittee, expressed strong commitment on the part of the relevant U.S. federal agencies for the process of developing DRIs.

Because the DRI reports contain an enormous amount of information about research recommendations and knowledge gaps, the steering committee called on the Food and Nutrition Board to gather the DRI research recommendations, synthesize them in a meaningful and useful database, and seek input from interested parties in completing the effort. This collaborative effort among federal agencies from the two countries and the Food and Nutrition Board was designed to facilitate the identification and response to important research needs. In turn, this effort will inform future studies of human nutrient requirements.

The steering committee's goals for the project include the following:

- Gather the research recommendations from the eight DRI reports
- Synthesize those recommendations in a searchable database
- Identify gaps in knowledge—including progress that has been made and the gaps that still need to be filled
- Stimulate research to fill gaps
- Assist sponsors in setting priorities
- Alert the research community to the gaps and priorities
- Make future DRI recommendations even more meaningful

Dr. Coates asked researchers and other users of the data contained in the DRI reports to provide the Federal DRI Steering Committee with suggestions for improving and making the most use out of the database of DRI research recommendations.

Canadian Involvement

Canada has been involved in the DRI process from its inception in the mid-1990s. In particular, Canada has contributed financial support, representatives of Canadian government agencies are participants in the Federal DRI Steering Committee, Canadian scientists have served on each of the DRI subcommittees and panels, and the Canadian government currently is funding the production of a summary volume of the

DRIs. This summary will be published in both French and English—the two official languages of Canada.

The DRIs have become the cornerstone of Canadian nutrition policies. Currently, they are being used in Canada for policy development, the setting of standards and regulations, conducting risk assessments, and providing advice to the Canadian population related to healthy eating. The Institute of Nutrition, Metabolism and Diabetes of the Canadian Institutes for Health Research is one of the sponsors of this workshop. This sponsorship demonstrates commitment to this effort by the major health research funding organization in Canada.

Several of the research gaps are of special concern to Canada. For example, information is required on how geographical variables affect the vitamin D needs of Canadians who have limited exposure to sunshine in the northern latitudes and on vitamin D status for various levels of intake throughout the life span. Moreover, additional information is needed on vitamin B_{12} requirements for the elderly and how these can be met. In Canada, currently, synthetic vitamin B_{12} is not approved for use in fortified foods. Thus, the only form of vitamin B_{12} that many elderly individuals can absorb is available only in the form of supplements. In developing policies on the fortification of foods, Canada relies on the DRIs for children for modeling purposes, but there are huge information gaps related to the nutrient requirements of children.

APPROACH AND FRAMEWORK OF THE DIETARY REFERENCE INTAKES

Presenter: John W. Erdman, Jr.

A Brief History of Recommended Dietary Allowances

The development and publication of nutrient recommendations in the United States officially began in the early 1940s with the first edition of *Recommended Dietary Allowances* (NRC, 1943). That first report, which was requested by the U.S. Department of Defense, yielded just 10 dietary recommendations: those for energy, protein, 2 minerals, and 6 vitamins. The intent of Recommended Dietary Allowances (RDAs) was to ensure adequate nutrition, especially protection from deficiency diseases, and to set standards for public health programs. Two major avenues provided the scientific basis of the RDAs: (1) observation of usual patterns that lead to healthy living, and (2) experimentally determined data on nutrient requirements.

The 10th (and final) edition of *Recommended Dietary Allowances* was published in 1989 (NRC, 1989b). By then, the scientific information base had expanded enough that the report contained recommendations for 7 minerals and 11 vitamins, in addition to protein and energy. In that report, Safe and Adequate Daily Dietary Intakes rather than RDAs were developed for an additional 2 vitamins and 5 minerals. These new nutrient values for 7 nutrients were ranges of the nutrients that were considered safe and adequate.

The users of RDAs included government, industry, academia, and health services. The uses of the RDAs, some of which were appropriate and some of which were not, included the following:

- Guide for procuring food supplies for groups of healthy persons
- Basis for planning meals for groups
- Reference point for evaluating the dietary intake of population subgroups
- Component of food and nutrition education programs
- Reference point for the nutrition labeling of food and dietary supplements

Development of a New Framework

In 1989, the National Research Council (NRC) released *Diet and Health* (NRC, 1989a), which focused on nutrients and dietary patterns as related to the reduction of chronic disease risk. Then, in the early 1990s, the Food and Nutrition Board addressed a number of concerns and issues related to establishing nutrient requirements and recommendations. Among these were

- a history of a lack of transparency for the process for establishing recommendations,
- little published information on how the recommended values were determined,
- new information on food components that had not been identified as nutrients (e.g., fiber and carotenoids),

- an evolving concern about nutrients' roles in protection against chronic disease,
- a number of new statistical approaches for examining data, and
- the use of the RDAs for some purposes that were considered to be inappropriate.

As a result, in 1993, the Food and Nutrition Board held a workshop called "How Should the Recommended Dietary Allowances Be Revised?" A report of the workshop was published the next year (IOM, 1994). That report proposed a new framework—the DRI framework. The framework included concepts of reduction of the risk of chronic diseases, a review of other dietary components, documentation of the rationale for the end points used, and recommendations to meet a variety of uses. It also included estimation of an upper intake level. Interest in setting upper levels grew, in part, because the new approach might increase recommendations for certain nutrients to alleviate chronic diseases, which, in turn, might move the intake values to a level that would be close to the upper level for one or more nutrients. Following release of the report of the workshop, the Food and Nutrition Board provided additional opportunities for input from scientists and users of nutrient recommendations.

Organizational Structure

The Food and Nutrition Board developed an organizational structure to carry out the DRI process, as shown in Figure 1-1. A standing committee oversaw the process, chaired for nearly seven years by the late Dr. Vernon Young. Two subcommittees were appointed to focus on specific aspects of the task—safe upper levels and applications of the DRIs. The Subcommittee on Upper Reference Levels of Nutrients provided input to the panels regarding safety and upper levels of intake, and the Subcommittee on Interpretation and Use of DRIs provided input to each panel concerning how to apply the DRIs for the nutrient group. Reflecting the joint nature of the project in the United States and Canada, Canadian and American scientists served on the committee, subcommittees, and panels.

Over time, six panels were appointed to address groups of nutrients. To some degree, nutrients were grouped together because of their relationship to chronic disease end points.

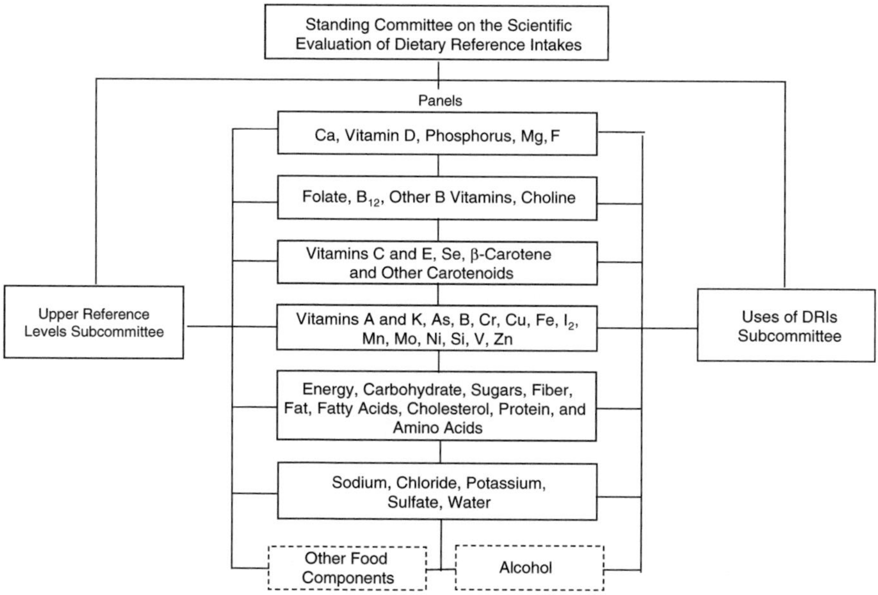

FIGURE 1-1 Organizational structure for the DRI process.
NOTE: Ca = calcium; Mg = magnesium; F = fluoride; Se = selenium; As = arsenic; B = Boron; Cr = chromium; Cu = copper; Fe = iron; I = iodine; Mn = manganese; Mo = molybdenum; Ni = nickel; Si = silicon; V = vanadium; Zn = zinc.

Types of DRI Values

The reports use four different types of DRI values:

1. Estimated Average Requirement (EAR)
2. Recommended Dietary Allowance (RDA)
3. Adequate Intake (AI)
4. Tolerable Upper Intake Level (UL)

With publication of the report on macronutrients, the Acceptable Micronutrient Distribution Range (AMDR) was added.

In Figure 1-2, three types of DRIs are placed on a hypothetical curve that depicts effects of increasing the observed level of intake. With a low level of intake, 100 percent of the population is deficient, based on some

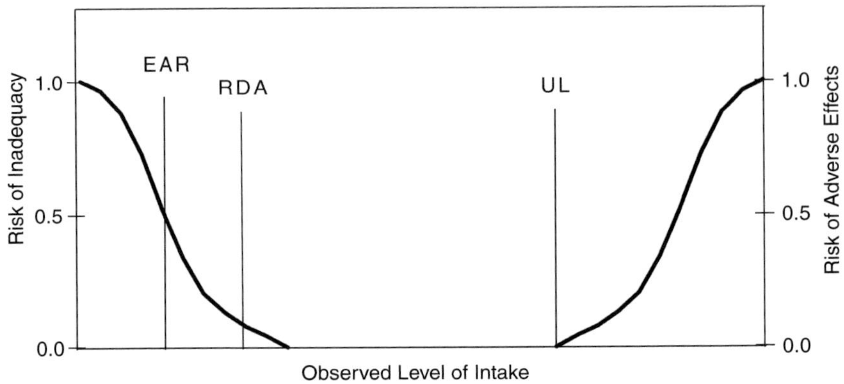

FIGURE 1-2 Relative positions of selected Dietary Reference Intake values on a curve showing intake versus risk.
NOTE: EAR = Estimated Average Requirement; RDA = Recommended Dietary Allowance; UL = Tolerable Upper Intake Level.

end-point criterion. With increasing intake, a point presumably would be reached at which 100 percent of the healthy population would have no deficiency or inadequacy based on that same end point.

The EAR is at the midpoint, where 50 percent of the population would meet the end-point criterion. The RDA, calculated as two standard deviations above the EAR,[2] is the intake level at which, theoretically, 97.5 percent of the population would meet that end-point criterion. AIs are set when data are insufficient to establish an EAR. The AI for a nutrient is a recommended average daily intake level based on observed or experimentally determined approximations or estimates of nutrient intake by a group (or groups) of apparently healthy people and is assumed to be adequate.

Notably, a chronic disease end point was used as the basis for the EAR or AI only for fluoride, potassium, total fiber, and for the AMDRs. Dr. Erdman commented that in 1993 and 1994, it was anticipated that a larger number of nutrients would use chronic disease end points. A chronic disease end point was used for the UL for sodium and chloride.

For some nutrients, ULs were set. ULs are defined as the highest level of daily nutrient intake that is likely to pose no risk of adverse health effects for almost all individuals in the specified life-stage group.

[2]This applies when the distribution of the requirement is assumed to be normal.

The adverse effect identified as a basis for a UL ranged from diarrhea to much more serious conditions.

The AMDRs include ranges of intakes of energy nutrients (protein, carbohydrates, and fats). These are ranges of macronutrient intakes that are associated with reduced risk of chronic disease while providing adequate intakes of essential nutrients for a given age and gender group. For adults, for example, the AMDR for fat is 20 to 35 percent of energy; for carbohydrate, it is 45 to 65 percent; and for protein it is 10 to 35 percent.

The DRI Reports

Based on the work of these committees and panels, the Institute of Medicine has published eight major DRI reports, as shown earlier in Box 1-1. For each report, the box also includes an abbreviated title; these abbreviated titles are used for convenience in the remainder of this workshop summary.

Closing

To close the introductory session, Dr. Erdman expressed appreciation for the broad support that has made it possible to produce the DRI reports. He also highlighted the upcoming single volume summary of the DRI reports, *Dietary Reference Intakes: The Essential Guide to Nutrient Requirements* (IOM, 2006a), and extended thanks to Canada for making the summary report possible. The format of the summary report is based on input from the intended audience—dietitians, nutritionists, and other health professionals—and the report is expected to be very useful for practitioners and those who teach them.

2

The Dietary Reference Intakes Research Synthesis Database[1]

Presenter: Janice Rice Okita

The database session provided a summary of the contents, features, and potential uses of the Dietary Reference Intakes (DRIs) Research Synthesis Database, which was still under development. The Food and Nutrition Board had been charged with entering all the research recommendations from the DRI reports into a database that would be searchable, user friendly, and widely available. Workshop participants were encouraged to test the database (www.iom.edu/DRIresearch2006) and provide feedback.

CONTENTS OF THE DRI RESEARCH SYNTHESIS DATABASE

The database contains more than 450 research recommendations—that is, all the research recommendations contained in eight DRI reports. For convenience, the database uses letters of the alphabet to identify the reports. In this workshop summary, each research recommendation has a number followed by a report identifier. For example, 29-A is a research recommendation from the report *Dietary Reference Intakes for Calcium, Phosphorus, Magnesium, Vitamin D, and Fluoride* (IOM, 1997). See Appendix D for a listing of the report identifiers.

Food and Nutrition Board staff categorized each of the research recommendations by key words to aid the search process. Staff members also are adding Medical Subject Heading (MeSH)[2] terms to the database,

[1]This chapter is based on a transcript and slides from the workshop.

[2]MeSH is the controlled vocabulary thesaurus of the U.S. National Library of Medicine, National Institutes of Health.

and the final version is expected to have full capability for users to search by the MeSH terms as well as by key words.

Review of the recommendations as a whole revealed that it would be helpful to categorize types of recommendations. In particular, staff used a two-tiered system that distinguishes "major knowledge gaps" from "knowledge gaps" (see Appendix D for criteria used). In addition, some of the research recommendations fit into a third category called "research methods." Examples include recommendations related to databases and nutrient assays.

Review of all the recommendations also made it apparent that it would be useful to identify cross-cutting topics. Obvious topics include age groups (e.g., adolescents, children, infants, elderly), biomarkers, dietary supplements, lactation and pregnancy, and the Tolerable Upper Intake Levels (ULs) and toxicity. Additional suggestions for cross-cutting topics would be welcome.

USE OF THE DATABASE

In developing the database, staff used two types of software—Excel and Access—both from Microsoft.[3] Each has advantages and disadvantages. Excel is widely available, many investigators use the software for a variety of purposes, and most users find data entry to be quite easy. However, Excel does not allow Boolean searches and has limited printing options. Access is less widely available, less familiar, and less user-friendly than is Excel. However, Access has a number of features that are highly desirable in a searchable database and that are not available in Excel. These features include capabilities to conduct tailored queries, save useful queries, and produce custom printouts of desired information.

To make the database as user-friendly as possible, staff placed two releases on the Institute of Medicine (IOM) website at www.iom.edu/DRIresearch2006 and sought feedback from users. The remainder of this chapter summarizes how to access and use the database. Additional information about the database appears in Appendix D.

[3]Microsoft Corporate Headquarters, Redmond, Washington.

ACCESSING AND USING THE DRI RESEARCH SYNTHESIS DATABASE

Entering www.iom.edu/DRIresearch2006 in the user's browser at the URL window accesses the Dietary Reference Intake Research Synthesis page of the IOM website. Clicking on DRI Research Synthesis Database accesses the database. The user then has a choice of downloading three files. One is a text file that provides some basic information on downloading and linking the files, lists the fields in the database, and provides some guidance for using the database.

The other two choices are for the two different forms of the database—one for use with Excel and the other for use with Access. The database is designed to be a desktop database—one that could be released as a compact disk (CD) or that could be downloaded from the IOM website. Upon downloading these files, the user can access them using the appropriate software.

Opening the Excel database gives the user a sense of the structure of the database. The columns include the number, ID code, recommendation, designation (type of recommendation), key words, and so on.

The Excel user might click on the column that contains all the recommendations. Alternatively the user could use the Find command to search for all the recommendations that contain the word *magnesium* (or any other word) in them. Searching on the key words column, the user sometimes obtains more recommendations than would be obtained by using the Find command to search for the same word in the recommendation. For example, if the user searches for biomarkers using the key words column, the listing will include recommendations containing the term *biological markers* as well as recommendations containing the word *biomarker*. Printing the list is not straightforward, however.

The Access file, but not the Excel file, can provide lists of the research recommendations by nutrient, by report, or by cross-cutting topic. Using Access, staff members have made it easy to obtain answers to common queries and to print the results in highly readable format. In particular, the Access research database includes more than 100 queries to cover each of the nutrients and some cross-cutting topics. For example, clicking on the saved query called "A-Calcium Report, All" sends a list of all the research recommendations in the DRI Calcium and Related Nutrients Report (IOM, 1997) to the computer monitor. Another example of a saved query is "Carotenoids List, Major." Clicking on this query sends a list of the major research recommendations pertaining to carotenoids. To see an example of a saved cross-cutting query, the user might want to look at a list of research recommendations pertaining to biomarkers or to infants.

To print the results of the query, the user clicks on Reports. More than 100 well-designed reports that correspond to the queries are available for printing. Appendix D provides a sample printout that shows the functionality of the database.

Users of the current release of the DRI Research Synthesis Database files were invited to submit comments and suggestions by August 1, 2006, so that they could be included in the final version. The intent has been to make the database easy to use and informative.

3

Dietary Reference Intakes for Calcium, Phosphorus, Magnesium, Vitamin D, and Fluoride[1]

Two university researchers presented information about Dietary Reference Intake (DRI) research recommendations contained in the Calcium and Related Nutrients Report (IOM, 1997). Bess Dawson-Hughes of Tufts University, who served on the panel for the report, highlighted a number of research recommendations that were considered to be of major importance for each of the five nutrients covered in the report and then made some comments about progress in those areas. Bruce W. Hollis of Medical University of South Carolina focused on the dietary requirement for vitamin D, which is his area of research.

DRI REPORT ON CALCIUM AND RELATED NUTRIENTS

Presenter: Bess Dawson-Hughes

Calcium

Major research recommendations for calcium included defining (1) the impact of calcium intake on mineral metabolism and peak bone mass; (2) genetic and calcium intake interactions; (3) the impact of calcium intake by adults on skeletal end points and on nonskeletal end points

[1]This chapter is an edited transcript of remarks and slides by Drs. Bess Dawson-Hughes and Bruce Hollis at the workshop. Comments made by Dr. Dawson-Hughes represent a composite of input from many of the panel members including Stephanie Atkinson, Steve Abrams, Robert Heany, Robert Rude, Connie Weaver, and Gary Whitford, and from James Penland (regarding magnesium).

such as blood pressure, cancer risk, and diabetes; and (4) the impact of calcium intake on the risk of developing a first or recurrent kidney stone.

The most notable progress is a much better understanding of the link between calcium intake and absorption, particularly in adolescents. In addition, data now relate some of the vitamin D polymorphisms to mineral metabolism in children. Information from Goulding and others (1998) indicates that milk intake in childhood influences fracture rates both in childhood and later in life in women.

The longest of several recent calcium intervention trials is a 7-year intervention study conducted by Matkovic et al. (2005). That study found that the bone mineral density of girls who were taller at the end of the 7-year interval benefited from supplementation. The results raise the question as to whether calcium intake should be set on the basis of body size, at least in children and adolescents.

Racial differences in bone turnover and calcium metabolism have been described. Over the last 9 years, numerous randomized controlled trials of adults have been published. The studies that had a placebo group with a low calcium intake and a reasonable level of compliance generally have shown beneficial effects of calcium supplementation on bone.

The Dietary Approaches to Stop Hypertension (DASH) Study has looked at dairy food intakes to reduce blood pressure. Several studies identify a small (3% to 5%) inverse effect of calcium on weight. That is controversial, but there seems to be a low-level association.

Data on the effect of high calcium intake on the occurrence of first kidney stone are now available from approximately 36,000 women in the Women's Health Initiative. Reportedly, a comprehensive analysis of the stone risk is underway. The report by Borghi et al. (2002) provides data on associations of calcium intake and recurring stones.

One recent 5-year calcium intervention trial (Prince et al., 2006) was conducted in western Australia. The trial included approximately 1,500 women with a mean age of 75 years. Usual calcium intakes averaged approximately 900 milligrams per day. This was a placebo-controlled trial in which the supplement provided 1,000 mg of calcium in the form of calcium carbonate. Table 3-1 shows that only about 57 percent of the subjects in the cohort had an adherence rate of 80 percent or higher. This actually is a fairly good degree of adherence for a very long intervention study. The subset of adherents had a statistically significant reduction in all fracture risk. Those in the intent-to-treat group had a similar trend, but it was not significant.

TABLE 3-1 Effect of 1,200 mg of Calcium Supplement Versus Placebo on Fracture Risk

	Percent of Subjects	Hazard Ratio [95% CI[a]]
All subjects	100%	0.87 [0.67–1.12]
Adherent subjects[b]	57%	0.66 [0.45–0.97]

[a]CI = confidence interval.
[b]Subjects maintaining an adherence rate of at least 80 percent.
SOURCE: Prince et al., 2006.

Vitamin D

Among the primary research recommendations for vitamin D are to (1) define optimal serum 25-hydroxyvitamin D [25-(OH)D] concentration according to age group, race, and latitude; and (2) define relationships between intake of vitamin D and serum 25-(OH)D.

The process of defining optimal vitamin D intake has been unfolding along the following lines over the last nine years. Three steps in the process are identifying the biological action affected by vitamin D, determining the amount of 25-(OH)D needed to optimize function for that biological action, and then defining the relationship between intake and serum 25-(OH)D.

Previously, parathyroid hormone (PTH) suppression was the primary gauge of optimum vitamin D status. Then, considerable development occurred in the biological action arena, particularly regarding musculoskeletal end points. Bone density, muscle performance, falls, and fractures now are key vitamin D musculoskeletal end points. A burgeoning area involves associations of vitamin D intake and 25-(OH)D with a wide variety of other very important end points, including the risk of developing diabetes, cancer, infection, periodontal disease, and osteoarthritis. These health problems involve a large proportion of the population.

A cross-sectional study out of Iceland, in over 900 individuals, examined the relative contributions of calcium and vitamin D to PTH suppression. Figure 3-1 shows that subjects were sorted by three categories of calcium intake, shown in the three types of bars and by categories of 25-(OH)D concentrations shown on the X axis. In persons with 25-(OH)D concentrations below 25 nmol/L, PTH was suppressed by increasing calcium intake. However, as the vitamin D concentration increases above 25 nmol/L, calcium plays a less obvious role in suppressing PTH. In Iceland, two-thirds of the people were at 25 nmol/L or more of 25-(OH)D, and in populations residing closer to the equator, one would expect to find a greater proportion with vitamin D concentrations greater than 25 nmol/L.

Table 3-2 lists vitamin D placebo-controlled intervention trials relevant to estimating the optimal 25-(OH)D concentration. The table includes the author, the dosage of vitamin D administered compared with placebo (some with calcium, some not), the 25-(OH)D concentration achieved on supplementation, and the changes in parathyroid hormone. It shows that four of the eight studies demonstrated a positive effect on nonvertebral fracture risk reduction. Based in part on these study results, many are estimating that a 25-(OH)D concentration of 75 nmol/L or higher will reduce the risk of fracture more than would lower concentrations of 25-(OH)D.

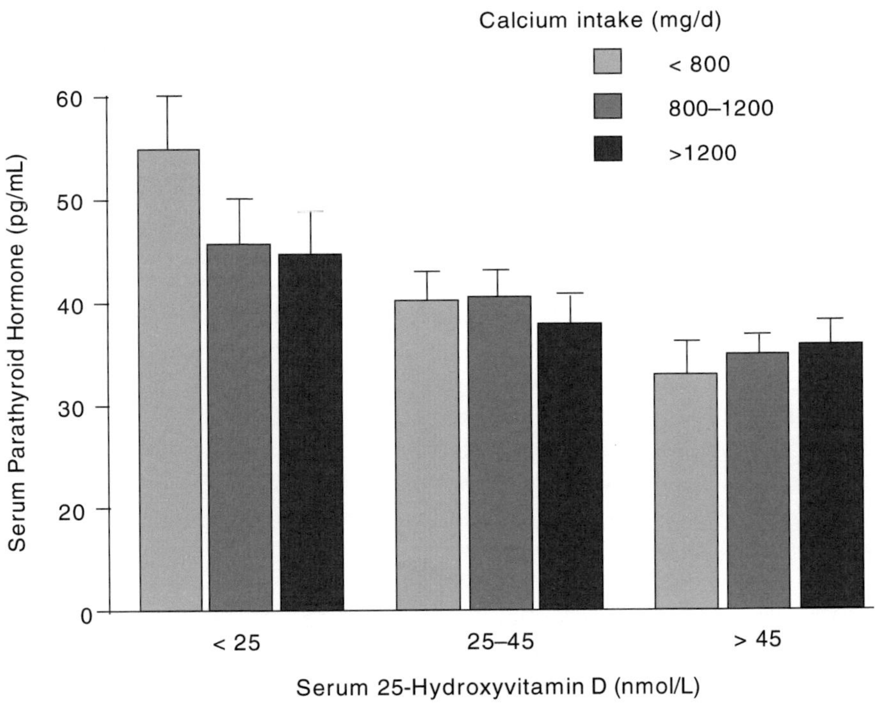

FIGURE 3-1 Serum parathyroid hormone concentration by serum 25-hydroxyvitamin D level and by level of calcium intake.
SOURCE: Steingrimsdottir et al. 2005. *JAMA*. 294: 2336-41. *Copyright© 2005, American Medical Association*. All rights reserved.

TABLE 3-2 Serum 25-Hydroxyvitamin D, Parathyroid Hormone, and Nonvertebral Fracture Responses to Supplementation with Vitamin D_3

Author, Year	Dose (IU/d)	25-(OH)D (nmol/L)	ΔPTH (%)	Effect on Nonvertebral Fracture
Chapuy et al., 2002	800	100	-47	+
Chapuy et al., 1992	800	100	-33	+
Dawson-Hughes et al., 1997	700	112	-28	+
Trivedi et al., 2003	820	74	?	+
Grant et al., 2005	800	63*	0	NS
Jackson et al., 2006	400	59*	?	NS
Lips et al., 1996	400	54	-6	NS
Meyer et al., 2002	400	64	?	NS

NOTE: ΔPTH = Change in parathyroid hormone concentration; NS = no statistically significant effect.

*Estimates in subsets of subjects.

It appears more useful to consider the 25-(OH)D concentration than the supplement dose. Take the case, for example, of the Randomized Evaluation of Calcium or Vitamin D (RECORD) Trial (Grant et al., 2005). The investigators gave the same dose of vitamin D as was given in many of the positive trials. Their compliance, however, was low: only half the subjects were taking any supplements at all at the 2-year mark into the 5-year trial. Consequently, the dose consumed could not have been as high as the amount being delivered.

Progress has been made regarding the safety of vitamin D. In a study involving daily dosing with either 1,000 or 4,000 IU of vitamin D per day over a 5-month period, no toxicity was invoked. In panel B (the 4,000 IU dose of vitamin D_3) in Figure 3-2, the mean serum 25-(OH)D concentration achieved was 100 nmol/L. Nearly all subjects were in the desired range of 75 to 80 nmol/L or higher. Although one subject's 25-(OH)D value rose to 138 nmol/L, that is a typical level for a person who works outdoors in the sun in the summertime. An average lifeguard will have a 25-(OH)D concentration of approximately 160 nmol/L. There is no sense of concern about the serum vitamin D concentrations shown in Figure 3-2.

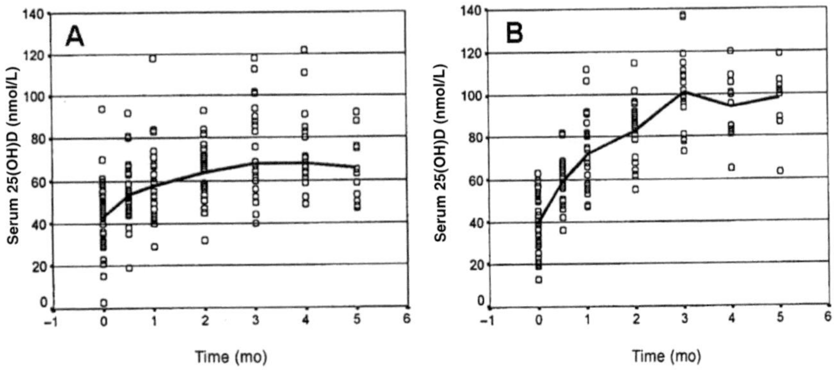

FIGURE 3-2 Serum 25-hydroxyvitamin D responses to two levels of vitamin D_3 supplementation over 6 months.
NOTE: A = 1,000 IU/d of vitamin D_3; B = 4,000 IU/d of vitamin D_3.
SOURCE: Veith et al. (2001). Reproduced with permission from *The American Journal of Clinical Nutrition.*

Data are just beginning to appear concerning vitamin D needs of children. However, much information still is needed, particularly for children in the age range of 6 months to 8 years. A very recent intervention study with 200 or 400 IU of vitamin D looked at the change in bone mineral content in young adolescent girls over a 1-year interval. Results showed step increases in the change in bone mineral content with more vitamin D supplementation.

For adults, more data are needed to refine estimates that 75 to 80 nmol/L of serum 25-(OH)D are needed for the musculoskeletal end points. There also is a great need to obtain threshold estimates for the chronic disease end points mentioned earlier. An enormous amount of work is being conducted in this area now.

Additional needs include standardization of 25-(OH)D assays and better quantitation of the vitamin D content of foods. For example, the vitamin D values for salmon (one of the main food sources of this vitamin) are based on wild salmon. Does farm salmon, which currently is widely consumed, have the same vitamin D content?

Phosphorus

For phosphorus, there were two key research recommendations: (1) for ages 1 to 18 years, to define the intake needed to optimize bone accretion; and (2) for children and adults, to define the relationship between phosphorus intake and the concentration of phosphorus in the blood.

Relatively little progress appears to have occurred in this area. Current identified research needs concern the potential problem of low phosphorus intake, especially by older individuals in the United States; the extent to which the increasing use of calcium supplements may decrease the bioavailability of phosphorus; and a potential increased need for phosphorus related to the introduction of anabolic agents for the treatment of osteoporosis.

Magnesium

The key research recommendations for magnesium were to (1) identify the magnesium intake needed for maximum accretion of bone in children and for preservation of bone in adults; (2) identify associations between magnesium intake and the development of other conditions such as hypertension, cardiovascular disease, and diabetes; and (3) identify and validate an accurate indicator of magnesium status.

Some interesting animal and epidemiological studies have been published recently, as mentioned briefly here. Rude and coworkers (2004, 2005, 2006) conducted several elegant magnesium depletion studies in rats. Table 3-3 shows that at half of the magnesium requirement, trabecular bone volume was decreased, and osteoclast number was higher. With further and further magnesium depletion, these effects became more exaggerated in the rats and, in addition, tumor necrosis factor-alpha concentrations rose. Unfortunately, parallel data in humans are unavailable.

TABLE 3-3 Magnesium Depletion and the Skeleton in Rats

Study	Diet, % Nutrient Requirement	Outcome
Rude et al., 2004	50	↓ Trabecular volume, ↑ osteoclast number
Rude et al., 2005	25	Also ↑ TNF-alpha
Rude et al., 2006	10	Also ↑ TNF-alpha

NOTE: TNF-alpha = tumor necrosis factor alpha

Two large epidemiologic studies involving large numbers of subjects with long follow-up periods are of special interest. In these studies, the subjects in the highest versus lowest quintile of magnesium intake had a decreased risk of developing both type II diabetes (Lopez-Ridaura et al., 2004) and stroke (Ascherio et al., 1998). Although these studies can help develop hypotheses that may be promising, the approach does not really isolate a nutrient—especially since the magnesium from food tends to be accompanied by other important nutrients.

Little has changed with regard to the indicators of magnesium status, but a report by Barbagallo and colleagues (2000) merits consideration. This study makes use of the facts that 99 percent of magnesium in the body is intracellular and that, of this, approximately 10 to 15 percent is in the ionized metabolically active form. These investigators found no differences in the free intracellular magnesium concentrations of normal subjects compared to hypertensive individuals or compared to persons with diabetes.

Fluoride

Key research recommendations for fluoride include (1) conducting epidemiologic research on habitual exposure to fluoride, particularly focusing on the prevention of dental caries, quality of bone, and the risk of developing fluorosis; and (2) identifying the factors that influence fluoride absorption and retention.

Two very comprehensive and important reports on fluoride were published over the last seven years—an epidemiologic study by Sowers et al. (2005) and another from the National Health and Nutrition Examination Survey (NHANES) by Beltran-Aguilar et al. (2005). The study by Sowers and colleagues had 4 years of follow-up and looked at fractures and changes in bone density in 1,300 women in three different communities in Iowa. The control community had a fluoride content of 1 ppm in the water supply (within the recommended level), and mean calcium intake was 754 mg/day. For comparison, one of the communities had the same fluoride content in the water but a high mean calcium intake (1,001 mg/day). The other test community had a high fluoride content (4 ppm) of the water, but calcium intake was comparable to that of the control community.

The bottom line is that the fracture rates were similar in the three communities. Bone densities were similar, with the exception of a minor increase in the forearm in the high fluoride community. These results do not raise much concern about fluoride in these communities.

Using NHANES data, Beltran-Aguilar et al. (2005) compared certain dental outcomes from the period of 1988–1994 with the same outcomes from 1999–2002. The investigators found that caries in permanent teeth in the United States have declined, as has tooth loss in older adults. The prevalence of enamel fluorosis has increased, however, starting in 1980. Racial and ethnic disparities persist in the prevalence of caries and enamel fluorosis.

THE DIETARY REQUIREMENT FOR VITAMIN D: LOOKING BEYOND BONE

Presenter: Bruce Hollis

This presentation focused on vitamin D. Dr. Hollis took the position that vitamin D_2 (the form of vitamin D obtained by the irradiation of ergocalciferol from plants) should be removed from use in food supplements and that vitamin D_3 (the form of the vitamin that is produced by the action of ultraviolet light on vitamin D precursors in the skin) should be used instead. The biggest reason given for this position is that vitamin D_2 is less biologically active than vitamin D_3 (Armas et al., 2004). Giving vitamin D_2 elicits more variable responses in 25-(OH)D values than does giving vitamin D_3.

Vitamin D_3 is metabolized fairly rapidly to 25-(OH)D, which is the major circulating form of vitamin D and is a biomarker for vitamin D status. One can influence the concentration of 25-(OH)D through diet or sun exposure, but one can have little influence on the amount of circulating 1,25-$(OH)_2$D—the active form of the vitamin. Vitamin D metabolism differs depending on the amount of vitamin D_3 supplied to the body. When vitamin D supplies are inadequate, the flow of 25-(OH)D through other potential pathways, including its utilization by peripheral tissues for paracrine regulation, is compromised. Dr. Hollis indicated that a chronic depleted status may be common today and that a depleted vitamin D status poses risks for within-tissue processing.

Research Questions on Vitamin D Requirements

Research on vitamin D requirements needs to consider the cutaneous generation of vitamin D and differences in vitamin D_3 generation that relate to skin color, latitude, the use of sun screen, and the amount of skin actually exposed to the sun. In view of the relative lack of vitamin D_3 in the food supply and public health recommendations to use sun screen to reduce the risk of skin cancer, what amount of oral vitamin D supplementation should be provided? Heaney et al. (2003) examined the response of 25-(OH)D as a function of oral vitamin D_3 intake over a 5-month period. Circulating 25-(OH)D values at the highest intakes (5,000 to 10,000 IU/day) were comparable to those resulting from extensive solar exposure, and those at the lowest intakes (400 to 1,000 IU/day) tended to decrease over time.

According to Dr. Hollis, the 400 IU (10 μg) dose of vitamin D supplied to subjects in the Women's Health Initiative studies was too small to increase the 25-(OH)D values at all. He based his position on the 2003 Heaney et al. study, including a regression of the equilibrium increment in serum 25-(OH)D concentration on the labeled dose for the mean intake by each treatment group.

Another important question involves the identification of optimal circulating concentrations of 25-(OH)D. Different types of evidence suggest that concentrations previously identified as normal are too low. In particular, Dr. Hollis noted problems with the interpretation of the study by Haddad and Chyu (1971) that identified a low 25-(OH)D level as normal. A biomarker would be especially useful if it would respond to both increases and decreases in the 25-(OH)D concentration.

Dr. Hollis indicated that effects of vitamin D on PTH are well known, as are vitamin D interactions in bone. He considers insulin sensitivity, beta cell function, immune function, circulating cytokines (both proinflammatory and anti-inflammatory), and cardiac health to be promising research areas.

There are several examples of relationships of vitamin D with infection. A recent study by Liu and colleagues (2006) provides an explanation for findings by Finsen (Rocchietta, 1960) that ultraviolet light benefits patients with lupus vulgaris and for the demonstrated beneficial effects of ultraviolet light exposure on tuberculosis patients in sanitoria. In particular, the study found that human toll-like receptor triggers a vitamin D receptor-dependent antimicrobial response. This response involves the innate immune system, which provides the first response to pathogens when they invade the body.

In Caucasians and African Americans, Liu and coworkers (2006) showed that nutritional vitamin D status controlled cathelicidin, an antimicrobial peptide made by monocytes and macrophages. At low concentrations (20 or 30 nmol/L) of serum 25-(OH)D, subjects could not mount a response to kill the internalized tuberculosis in the macrophages. After supplementation with vitamin D in amounts sufficient to achieve serum 25-(OH)D concentrations of 80 nmol/L, the subjects could mount this attack, produce cathelicidin, and attack the tuberculosis.

A brief study conducted in India (Rehman, 1994) shows that vitamin D supplements of 60,000 IU/week for 6 weeks could help children with elevated alkaline phosphatase concentrations to overcome respiratory infections.

A study by Giovannucci and colleagues (2006) estimates the effects of a 25-nmol/L increase in serum 25-(OH)D in a population on the odds ratios of developing various forms of cancer. For 11 of the 14 forms of cancer, the odds ratios of developing those cancers are less than one. Additional work is in progress.

A small pilot vitamin D supplementation study (Wagner et al., 2006) looked at periodic changes in maternal and infant blood concentrations of 25-(OH)D and of vitamin D activity in mother's milk. The study found that the higher level of maternal vitamin D_3 supplementation (6,400 IU compared with 400 IU) resulted in substantial increases in vitamin D_3 and 25-(OH)D in the mother and in milk vitamin D activity. The serum 25-(OH)D concentration in the infants of the highly supplemented women was comparable to that of infants who were supplemented directly.

Dr. Hollis challenged the current Adequate Intake (AI) of 10 μg of vitamin D/day for adults and probably for adolescents as not supportive of health. He stated that it is almost certain that chronic deficiency of vitamin D puts populations at risk for debilitating chronic diseases. Moreover, he posited that a serum concentration of 80 nmol/L of 25-(OH)D, which has been proposed to protect the skeleton, is too low to reduce the risk of muscular sclerosis or cancer or to promote immune function.

Tolerable Upper Intake Level for Vitamin D

Dr. Hollis challenged the Tolerable Upper Intake Level (UL) that the Institute of Medicine set for vitamin D. In studies by Hollis and Wagner (2004), Wagner et al. (2006), and Heaney et al. (2003) involving 10,000 IU/day of vitamin D (or more), no instances of hypercalciuria or hypercalcemia occurred. Furthermore, Dr. Hollis indicated that the low UL is an impediment to human health because it sets too low a limit on what the vitamin manufacturers can add to their vitamin supplements.

DISCUSSION

Questions and comments by Drs. Dennis Bier, Irwin Rosenberg, Larry Appel, Paul Pencharz, and Robert Russell are summarized below, along with responses from the presenters.

Optimal Parathyroid Hormone level

Dr. Bier asked how one defines the optimal PTH level in the context of adequacy. Drs. Hollis and Dawson-Hughes responded that many sound studies with reliable PTH assays have looked at this relationship. They all indicate that one can suppress PTH serially only until the 25-(OH)D concentration reaches approximately 80 nmol/L. Lower rates of bone loss provide the basis for the suppression. Neither calcium nor vitamin D (nor both) can suppress PTH more than a maximum of 80 to 90 percent. In such studies, the calcium range is defined in the usual way, with a group of healthy individuals.

Circular Argument

Dr. Bier expressed concern about issues related to PTH suppression and about a circular argument relating to the reference range for calcium. In particular, the reference range for calcium was said to be defined by values obtained from a group of "healthy individuals," but presentations pointed out the high prevalence of inadequate vitamin D in the population, which presumably is not healthy. Dr. Hollis responded that some recent studies address the points of having an adequate calcium index and setting the PTH reference ranges in relation to adequate vitamin D status.

Measures of Early Adverse Effects

Dr. Rosenberg asked what are potential measures of early adverse effects. Dr. Dawson-Hughes responded that probably the easiest and least expensive measure to obtain would be a random spot-urine calcium, which correlates very highly with the 24-hour urine calcium-to-creatinine ratio. That correlation is so strong that one would not need to conduct a 24-hour urine collection to assess safety. Basically, the random spot-urine calcium content would increase before the renal threshold was exceeded and before an increase in the blood calcium concentration occurred. Thus, the random spot-urine calcium would be an early point for detection, and it would be easier to interpret than a PTH value. Such a measurement would not be used to set a requirement but to monitor for safety. Dr. Hollis agreed that the random spot-urine calcium could be measured easily in a research setting or a clinical setting. He added that, because PTH is potentially cardiotoxic, it probably is in the interest of cardiovascular health to have lower PTH concentration as well. Dr. Dawson-Hughes stated that there is no evidence of any extension of the curve of the inverse relationship between insufficient levels of either calcium or vitamin D intake and PTH concentration.

Vitamin D and Chronic Illness

Dr. Hollis suggested that lack of vitamin D might be related to the high prevalence of lupus, multiple sclerosis, and diabetes among a population of African Americans called the Gullah in South Carolina. He reported that their vitamin D concentrations were the lowest he had ever seen.

Clarification of Units

Dr. Bier asked about the dramatic increase in maternal vitamin D intake that had a relatively small effect on circulating 25-(OH)D concentrations for the mother and the baby—the circulating levels for the mother and the infant were still below 80. Dr. Hollis clarified that the units are nanograms. To convert nanograms to nanomoles, one multiplies that number times 2.5.

Maternal-Infant Findings

Dr. Pencharz referred to a Muslim woman who bore a baby with neonatal rickets. These investigators in Saudi Arabia were able to treat the neonatal rickets by having the mother exposed to sunlight. That proved in a biological way what Dr. Hollis has shown biochemically. It appears that the evidence now supports recommendations to supplement the mother. Dr. Hollis responded that blinded maternal studies are underway but the increased blood concentrations of 25-(OH)D clearly indicate the individuals who are receiving the vitamin D. Data still are needed.

A model of the transfer of vitamin D during lactation is evolving. In response to questions from Dr. Allen, Dr. Hollis indicated that about 0.5 percent of the circulating 25-(OH)D passes into breast milk but that 30 to 80 percent of the parent compound (vitamin D_3) passes into the milk.

Persistence of Circulating 25-(OH)D

Dr. Russell asked how long very high blood concentrations of 25-(OH)D persist after extensive sun exposure, as in a lifeguard working outside. Dr. Dawson-Hughes was unaware of such data but referred to data from healthy older subjects in Boston. In the summer, their concentration of 25-(OH)D is approximately 80, and it decreases to about 60 in the winter. Dr. Hollis stated that the half life of 25-(OH)D is approximately 3 weeks.

Vitamin D_2 Versus D_3

Dr. Whiting asked Dr. Dawson-Hughes to elaborate on the relative value of vitamin D_2 and D_3. Dr. Dawson-Hughes responded that, from the current available evidence, D_3 is preferred. Although the evidence base is not extensive, it is consistent in suggesting that, for a given dose of D_2 or D_3, over at least a 2-week period, a considerably larger increment in the total 25-(OH)D concentration occurs with repeated dosing with vitamin D_3.

The study by Armas and colleagues (2004), which used a single dose of 50,000 units of vitamin D_2 or D_3, found similar increments in 25-(OH)D over the first 3 days; but subsequently the total 25-(OH)D concentration decreased in the D_2-treated subjects. In fact, it was lower than baseline at the end of 30 days. In contrast, the concentration in the D_3-treated subjects remained well above the baseline level at 30 days. Thus, the staying power of the single dose of vitamin D_3 is greater, and the increment over 2 weeks is greater. Vitamin D_2 can be effective, but it takes a much larger dose on a frequently repeated dosing regimen.

4

Dietary Reference Intakes for Thiamin, Riboflavin, Niacin, Vitamin B_6, Folate, Vitamin B_{12}, Pantothenic Acid, Biotin, and Choline[1]

In the presentations on the B Vitamins and Choline Report (IOM, 1998a), Steven H. Zeisel of the University of North Carolina–Chapel Hill (former member of the Panel on B Vitamins and Choline) addressed research on thiamin, riboflavin, niacin, pantothenic acid, and choline.[2] Dr. Patrick Stover of Cornell University covered folate, vitamins B_{12} and B_6, and biotin. Both presenters addressed lack of progress and new developments since 1997–1998, and they suggested future topics for research.

DISCUSSION OF RESEARCH RECOMMENDATIONS: THIAMIN, RIBOFLAVIN, NIACIN, PANTOTHENIC ACID, AND CHOLINE

Presenter: Steven H. Zeisel

This presentation highlighted major new developments, pointed out that genetic polymorphism and epigenetics merit special attention, and addressed major research gaps and the progress made.

---

[1]This chapter was prepared from the workshop transcript and slides.

[2]Dr. Zeisel's summary for the nutrients was based on calls to experts, recent reviews, and checking recent articles appearing in PubMed.

Major New Developments

Genetic Polymorphisms

New science in genetic polymorphisms suggests that the requirements for some of the nutrients vary, in part dependent on whether individuals possess single nucleotide polymorphisms (SNPs). SNPs are deoxyribonucleic acid (DNA) sequence variations that occur when a single nucleotide (A, T, C, or G) in the genome sequence is altered. Such genetic polymorphisms are not rare.

In setting Recommended Dietary Allowances (RDAs), the Panel on B Vitamins and Choline assumed that it had to cover only 95 percent of the population and that it did not need to address genetic mutations. For some of these nutrients, however, more than half the population has at least one genetic polymorphism. Thus, genetic mutations merit attention.

Epigenetics

The area of epigenetics has developed tremendously since the B Vitamins and Choline Report was written. Clearly, some of the nutrients in this group, specifically the methyl donors and biotin, are part of the process of epigenetic modification. Considerable data point to the need to consider whether gene expression is being changed by changes made to the promoter regions of genes or to the histones that surround genes.

Major Research Gaps and Progress Made

Major research gaps identified in the report included (1) human information on the requirements of children, pregnant and lactating women, and the elderly; (2) other indicators that could be used to assess function; and (3) adverse effects of high doses of the nutrient. A summary follows of progress made with regard to thiamin, riboflavin, niacin, pantothenic acid, and choline.

Thiamin

Little has been done to meet the research needs pertaining to thiamin.

Riboflavin

Since 1998, at least one large population study (O'Brien et al., 2001) on intake reports that a sizable segment of the population (12.5 percent of men and 20.6 percent of women) had intakes below the Estimated Average Requirement (EAR) in Ireland.

Hustad and coworkers (2000) show that riboflavin is inversely associated with homocysteine concentration in blood. The authors propose that individuals who have a SNP in the flavin-requiring enzyme methylene tetrahydrofolate reductase (MTHFR) are sensitive to riboflavin concentrations. With higher intakes of riboflavin, the homocysteine concentration in their blood decreases.

Flavin-adenine dinucleotide (FAD)-dependent glutathione reductases have been used as the markers for riboflavin sufficiency in setting the EAR for riboflavin. Some work suggests a new functional measure for riboflavin status. In particular, a clinical trial (Jacques et al., 2005) reports a reduction of age-related lens opacification in humans treated with riboflavin supplements. Cataract production was an end point that was not fully considered when setting the EAR for riboflavin, but it probably is of interest in the consideration of revisions to riboflavin requirements.

Niacin

Research gaps Research gaps particular to niacin include (1) increased niacin requirements secondary to oxidant exposure, (2) the identification of a better method for determining niacin status other than the urinary excretion currently used, and (3) improvement of nutrient databases to differentiate the forms of niacin—specifically the naturally occurring niacin content of foods and niacin added as a fortificant.

Progress made Some progress has been made in addressing niacin research gaps since 1998:

- A toxicology panel was convened; in 2005, it reported on the toxicity and potential toxicity of higher dose niacin (Cosmetic Ingredient Review Expert Panel, 2005). That report discusses possible end points and markers, and it would be useful in reconsidering Tolerable Upper Intake Levels (ULs) for niacin.

- High and low affinity nicotinic acid receptors have been identified and cloned (Wise et al., 2003).
- A G-protein-coupled receptor, HM74A, has been shown to mediate skin flushing (a side effect of high niacin intake) (Benyo et al., 2005). The G-protein-coupled receptor might be used to define niacin status and the niacin requirement in terms of another functional end point—namely, the activation or inactivation of that receptor.
- Results of numerous studies have been published on the pharmacological use of niacin for the reduction of hyperlipidemia. Two are especially notable: (1) the Atherosclerotic Disease Multiple Intervention Trial (ADMIT), a randomized controlled trial in patients with diabetes and peripheral artery disease; and (2) the Arterial Biology for the Investigation for the Treatment Effects of Reducing Cholesterol (ARBITER) trial, a double-blind, placebo-controlled style of extended-release niacin. With regard to the DRIs, both of those trials probably are most useful for defining human exposure and potential toxicity at high doses. However, they might also be useful in defining peripheral vascular disease function as an end point for niacin optimization.

Pantothenic Acid

Although lack of pantothenic acid has been seen to cause deficiency in humans very rarely, this vitamin is a widely used cofactor. Very little information was available about pantothenic acid in 1998, and more recent information has been provided by only two studies—both of which address assays for pantothenic acid in beverages, vitamins, and foods. Improved assay methods might help to improve the estimates of pantothenic acid content in food composition databases.

Choline

In 1998, insufficient data were available to set an EAR for choline, so Adequate Intakes (AIs) were set instead. Major research gaps particular to choline included its roles in chronic disease, bioavailability, metabolic effects, and interrelationships with vitamins B_{12} and B_6 and with methionine and folate metabolism. Choline has three functions: methyl donation, lipid formation, and formation of acetyl choline. Could methyl donors spare the entire requirement for choline or not?

All the studies that had been done before 1998 used male subjects. Because data on the choline content of foods were very sparse, the panel had little information on the choline content of the food supply or the extent of human exposure to choline. Limited data were available concerning high pharmacological doses of choline and their side effects; these data were used to establish a UL.

Depletion–repletion study findings New human data obtained from a 92-day depletion–repletion study (da Costa et al., 2006a,b) demonstrate that estrogen induces the endogenous synthesis of choline. Eighty percent of men and postmenopausal women developed liver and muscle dysfunction when deprived of choline, but only 44 percent of premenopausal women did.

At baseline, 60 individuals were given 550 mg of choline per 70 kg of body weight daily for 10 days (see Figure 4-1). Individuals then were depleted (given less than 50 mg/per 70 kg of body weight daily) until they developed signs of deficiency or for a maximum of 42 days. Fifty-five percent of women with estrogen did not need any choline for 42 days. Although their blood concentrations decreased, they did not develop other signs of choline depletion. Individuals who developed organ dysfunction were given graded doses of choline until they reverted to normal. Liver dysfunction (i.e., fatty liver by mass resonance imaging) was the common sign of depletion.

A subgroup of the individuals developed muscle dysfunction, as identified by creatine phosphokinase leakage into the plasma, which resolved with the refeeding of choline. This outcome affected 10 percent of the population, including men and one postmenopausal woman. Other research indicates that some men require substantially more than the current AI for choline (da Costa et al., 2006a). Potential functional markers for choline include muscle damage, lymphocyte apoptosis, and elevated homocysteine after a methionine load.

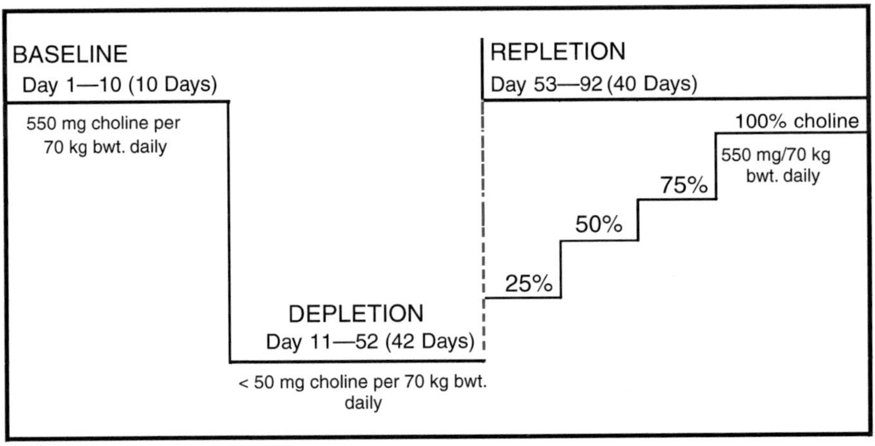

FIGURE 4-1 Study design for choline depletion–repletion trial. The trial included 31 healthy men and 35 health women. The daily baseline diet also contains 400 dietary folate equivalents (DFE) and the depletion and repletion diets have 100 DFE. On Day 11, subjects are randomized to 100 DFE (placebo) or 400 μg folic acid for the remainder of the study.
NOTE: bwt. = body weight.
SOURCE: da Costa et al. (2006b). Reproduced with permission from *The American Journal of Clinical Nutrition.*

The finding that premenopausal women are less likely to develop organ dysfunction when fed a low choline diet led to the examination of the gene that encodes for the enzyme that allows the liver to make the choline moiety. That gene has a number of estrogen-response elements in its promoter, and it is induced by estrogen. Further investigation revealed that individuals who develop organ dysfunction when deprived of choline have a greatly increased risk if they have one or two of several genetic polymorphisms in genes of choline or folate metabolism. The study found a polymorphism in phosphatidylethanolamine-*N*-methyltransferase (PEMT), the gene responsible for endogenous biosynthesis of the choline moiety.

The women who have this SNP in the PEMT promoter have increased susceptibility to choline deficiency (which is characterized by fatty liver, muscle and liver damage) with an observed risk 25 times that of controls. This huge increase in observed risk made it possible to identify the risk with only 60 subjects in this clinical study. A SNP in the gene for methyl-tetrahydrofolate dehydrogenase 1 (MTHFD1) also increased observed risk for developing choline deficiency (Kohlmeier et al., 2005).

Of particular note is that the SNPs related to choline deficiency are not rare. For example, 18 percent of subjects were homozygous for the PEMT SNP, and more than half the population has one allele for this SNP.

Food composition data and epidemiologic findings Several epidemiologic studies have examined associations of choline intake with health-related outcomes. These studies were possible because new food composition data on choline are available in tables from the U.S. Department of Agriculture (USDA).

In a case-control study, Shaw and coworkers (2004) found that women in the lowest quartile for dietary choline intake who also have a low dietary intake of folate have four times the risk of having a baby with a neural tube defect than mothers who are in the highest quartile of choline intake. More recently, Shaw and colleagues (2006) reported that the risk for cleft lip and palate in the high choline intake group is half that of the low choline intake group.

A large epidemiologic study reported an inverse relationship between dietary choline intake and plasma total homocysteine concentration (Cho et al., 2006). An intervention trial demonstrated that treatment with betaine, which is a choline metabolite, reduces the homocysteine concentration in humans (Melse-Boonstra et al., 2005).

Concluding Remarks

Dr. Zeisel ended his presentation by suggesting that future DRI panels address the roles of genetic polymorphisms when revising DRIs and that researchers consider conducting studies to determine whether there is a differential response, based on SNPs, to classical depletion–repletion.

DISCUSSION OF RESEARCH RECOMMENDATIONS

Presenter: Patrick J. Stover

Biotin

The one major gap listed for biotin was a serious lack of data to determine an EAR. The gap exists because biotin deficiency is extremely rare. Data suggest that humans obtain most of their biotin from microflora in the gut.

Among the new discoveries is the finding that biotin modifies histones (Stanley et al., 2001). It has been known for years that biotin affects the expression of enzymes in carbohydrate metabolism; the modification of histones and chromatin by biotin is an epigenetic signature that probably accounts for these findings. This finding also was confirmed with the identification of holocarboxylase synthase deficiency. This deficiency results in decreased histone biotinylation (Narang et al., 2004) and in neurological development and/or metabolic abnormalities that can be resolved with pharmacological levels of biotin. These genomic effects may provide new indicators for setting an EAR for biotin.

Vitamin B_6

Major research gaps listed for vitamin B_6 (pyridoxine) include better indicators for the requirement and information about genetic variation, chronic disease prevention, interaction with other vitamins, and the needs of children, the elderly, and pregnant and lactating women. Relatively little progress has been made.

Perhaps the biggest recent discovery was the confirmation that the plasma vitamin B_6 concentration falls dramatically in inflammation (Chiang et al., 2005b; Gori et al., 2006; Younes-Mhenni et al., 2004). Vitamin B_6 concentration is inversely correlated with C-reactive protein (CRP) and interleukin-6 (IL-6) in a number of disorders, including sickle cell, Crohn's disease, and rheumatoid arthritis. Pyridoxine supplementation has been shown to correct the deficiencies in some of these states, but not the inflammation (Chiang, 2005a).

These findings may have bearing on the UL. The loss of vitamin B_6 in inflammation is not due to urinary excretion; rather the vitamin B_6 is sequestered somewhere in the body. The lowering of plasma vitamin B_6 concentration may be a protective homeostatic response to inflammation. If demonstrated, this may indicate the potential for unidentified adverse effects resulting from pyridoxine supplementation.

Folate

Progress in Filling Research Gaps

A summary of progress in filling research gaps on folate appears below. Folic acid is a synthetic form of folate that is not normally found in foods—a form that can be converted to a natural form of folate once ingested.

Effects of folic acid fortification The mandatory fortification of enriched cereal grains with folic acid, which began in the United States in the late 1990s, has provided the opportunity for comprehensive analysis of risks and benefits of folic acid fortification. Good data are available on the substantial reduction of the incidence of neural tube defects that occurred following this mandatory fortification. Investigators are still examining data on effects of the fortification on conditions such as vascular disease, cancer, cognition outcomes, and dementia.

Genetic variants New genetic variants have been identified that affect carbon metabolism and that are risk factors for various disease outcomes. In addition to the MTHFR polymorphism known before 1998, researchers have identified another risk factor for neural tube defects, the MTHFD1 polymorphism, which was mentioned by Dr. Zeisel in relation to choline deficiency. Although these two human polymorphisms in folate metabolism are associated with increased risk for neural tube defects and alter one-carbon metabolism, they make up only a small fraction of the total genetic component that poses risk for neural tube defects.

Concern had been raised about whether the EARs for folate cover individuals with MTHFR polymorphism. This type of polymorphism is common—homozygotes for this population represent about 20 percent of the Caucasian and Asian populations. A recent depletion–repletion study (Guinotte et al., 2003) demonstrated that the current RDA for folate is adequate for young women for all three MTHFR phenotypes, suggesting that there is not a need for individualized requirements.

Potential indicator of folate requirement Preliminary data from the Third National Health and Nutrition Examination Survey (NHANES III) indicate that a useful cut point appears when homocysteine concentration is graphed against serum folate. Thus, a serum folate concentration of 10 nmol/L could serve as a useful indicator for the folate requirement.

Bioavailability Relatively little research has been conducted on the bioavailability of folate. Despite several studies, the interaction of folate with vitamin B_{12} deficiency remains to be determined. The concern is that adequate folate or high intake of folate may exacerbate the neurological symptoms and neurodegeneration associated with vitamin B_{12} deficiency, but this notion has yet to be proven or dismissed.

Folate requirements for infants and other special groups Most of the work related to the role of folate in the differentiation of development is still descriptive, not mechanistic. Little progress has been made in determining whether folate requirements vary by trimester in pregnancy or in obtaining data specific to folate requirements for children, elderly persons, and women of reproductive age.

Interactions with other nutrients Considerable data are available now regarding interactions of folate with certain other B vitamins and choline, both of which affect methylation status—especially the methylation of DNA and histones, which has effects on gene expression and stem cell programming.

Measurement of folate In analytical methodology, the biggest advancements have been made in the area of developing mass spectrometry techniques to measure folate concentration in serum.

New Concern

Among persons who have high intakes of folic acid, the unmetabolized form may appear in serum (Kelly et al., 1997; Troen et al., 2006). Seventy-eight percent of fasting adult participants in one study exhibited the presence of a substantial concentration of unmetabolized folic acid in serum. Concern has been raised about this—with regard both to children and adults. Folic acid itself is not a biologically active form of the vitamin, and it can have inhibitory properties. Troen and colleagues (2006) showed reduced natural killer cell cytotoxicity in women with folic acid present in the plasma.

Vitamin B_{12}

Major gaps related to vitamin B_{12} included

- its role in vascular disease;
- the impact of genetic variation;
- requirements in the elderly (one in six individuals over the age of 65 years is believed to be at risk for deficiency of vitamin B_{12});
- the effect of folate on progression of clinical symptoms of vitamin B_{12} deficiency, especially neurological outcomes;
- methods to detect status;
- indicators, especially in the elderly and vegans who have a propensity to become vitamin B_{12} deficient; and
- the efficacy of vitamin B_{12} fortification, should such fortification be initiated.

A polymorphism in transcarbolamine 2 has been found to affect indicators of blood B_{12} status, namely holotranscobalamin (holoTC concentration) and homocysteine concentration. Some progress has occurred in developing methods to determine vitamin B_{12} status: a holoTC kit is now available and may be an improvement, and other diagnostic kits are being developed.

Better indicators may also be available. In particular, the serum B_{12} value required to maintain hematological status (estimated earlier to be 150 pmol/L of serum B_{12}) is consistent with cut points for the log of homocysteine and the log of methyl-malonic acid versus serum B_{12} that occur near 150 pmol/L of serum B_{12} (Unpublished data, Jacob Selhub, Tufts University, 2006).

Future Perspectives

In terms of future perspectives, Dr. Stover focused on three areas: (1) disease and pathology outcomes, (2) genetic variation and requirements, and (3) fetal/stem cell programming.

Disease and Pathology Outcomes

MTHFR polymorphism inhibits the remethylation cycle, which may increase the homocysteine concentration of the blood, decrease methylation potential, and alter chromatin structure and gene expression. These alterations in biochemistry present both benefits and risks. For example, in utero risk for neural tube defects increases, as does the risk for miscarriage; but homozygous carriers of that polymorphism have a 70 percent reduction in risk for colon cancer compared to people who carry the more prevalent allele. This raises the question of whether a given nutrient intake level presents opposing benefits and risks for different diseases.

An increasing literature raises concern that a high folate status actually may present risk for colon cancer. That is, folate may be preventive in the initiation stage of cancers, but it may accelerate cellular transformation once the cancer is initiated. Thus, great care is needed in choosing outcomes on which to base the DRIs.

Genetic Variation and Requirements

With regard to genetic variation and requirements, it will be important to assess whether or not to individualize dietary requirements to subgroups that have a specific genetic polymorphism. In doing so, it is necessary to consider both the penetrance of the polymorphism (that is, the probability of expressing a phenotype from the given genotype at a given time) and its prevalence (which is a measure of the proportion of persons in the population with a certain SNP at a given time).

Evidence suggests that few SNPs are likely to be sufficiently penetrant to warrant genotype-specific recommendations. One basis for this position is that most of the SNPs known that affect indicators of status, at least in B vitamin metabolism, also are risk factors for miscarriage. The current experience indicates that genotypes that confer large differences in nutrient utilization and hence nutritional requirements will probably be lost in utero. However, some have suggested that the use of supplemental folate reduces rates of human spontaneous abortion. That is, given that folate apparently can prevent neural tube defects, it might rescue some of these miscarriages. The desirability of increasing disease alleles in the population is an open question and probably warrants some attention.

SNP–SNP interactions are likely to be more penetrant than most SNPs in isolation, but they have a lower prevalence. In general, as the penetrance of an SNP or SNP–SNP interaction increases, in terms of the effects of genetics on an indicator of status or outcome, the prevalence of that genetic variation decreases.

Examples of gene–gene interactions from Dr. Stover's laboratory involve cytoplasmic serine hydroxymethyltransferase (cSHMT) and 5-MTHFR. Results from the National Aging Study cohort analysis (Lim et al., 2005) show that neither the MTHFR polymorphism or the cSHMT polymorphism is very penetrant in terms of the risk of cardiovascular disease. However, cardiovascular disease risk increases if cSHMT polymorphism occurs among heterozygotes for the MTHFR polymorphism. Moreover, for homozygotes with both of the polymorphisms, the risk increases substantially. Thus, gene–gene interactions are important, but they have low prevalence.

Dr. Stover suggested the development of a framework for establishing impacts and cut-off points for genetic variation that addresses two major points: (1) How prevalent do these polymorphisms have to be to warrant genotype specific recommendations? and (2) What is the penetrance—that is, what is the genetic contribution of variation compared to the overall variation in requirement—and is that penetrance sufficient to warrant the use of genotypic-specific results to develop nutrient recommendations for subgroups?

Fetal and Stem Cell Programming

Dr. Stover emphasized the importance of investigating fetal and stem cell programming, which first received attention by the nutrition community related to Barker's fetal origins of adult disease hypothesis. This hypothesis suggests that fetal environmental exposures, especially nutrition, act in utero or in the neonate to program risk for adult health outcomes.

Evidence from mouse models suggests that folate can program gene expression (Cooney et al., 2002; Dolinoy et al., 2006; Morgan et al.,

1999; Waterland and Jirtle, 2003) A number of mouse models involve a genetic deletion that results either in nonviable embryos or some sort of a severe phenotype that can be rescued with nutrition. Thus, care is warranted related to the possibility that epigenetic effects modify genetic insults that exist in the human population. Dr. Stover believes that certain reprogramming events probably are common, can be modified by nutrition, and influence a number of folate-associated diseases.

Concluding Remarks

In conclusion, Dr. Stover emphasized the need to consider genetic variation, determine relevant parameters, and determine whether or not *individual* recommendations for B vitamin requirements are needed. Furthermore, there is a need for better understanding of epigenetic effects. In investigating new indicators for both the EAR and UL, a disease prevention approach could involve targeting the molecular antecedents of disease. Promising ones might include molecular antecedents for cancer and for other diseases with mutation rates that can be measured in the population. However, since this approach probably would result in increasing the RDA, attention also would need to be given to new concerns for ULs, including epigenetic effects and genetic rescue.

DISCUSSION

A number of comments made during the discussion relate to the DRI paradigm. Those comments appear at the end of Chapter 13, “Wrap-Up.”

Dr. Appel asked about homocysteine as a surrogate for folate intake. In particular, findings in recently published clinical trials indicated that decreases in serum homocysteine concentration were not accompanied by a reduction in adverse health outcomes. In some cases, there was the appearance of potential harm. Considering this, how could homocysteine serve as a useful surrogate for folate intake? Dr. Stover responded that those findings were from secondary prevention trials and that primary prevention trials are needed because that probably is where homocysteine is exerting its effects.

5

Dietary Reference Intakes for Vitamin C, Vitamin E, Selenium, and Carotenoids[1]

Presentations on the Dietary Reference Intakes (DRI) Antioxidants Report (IOM, 2000b) were given by Susan Taylor Mayne of Yale University School of Medicine, who served on the panel for the report, and by John N. Hathcock of the Council for Responsible Nutrition, who was asked to provide a fresh perspective. Dr. Mayne provided an overview of progress made and addressed emerging or persistent questions. (Vitamin C was not covered because of time limitations.) She also addressed consistency of the research recommendations with public health concerns, methods to address research recommendations in future DRIs, and the use of Adequate Intakes (AIs). Dr. Hathcock's presentation focused on the DRI process.

DISCUSSION OF RESEARCH RECOMMENDATIONS: VITAMIN C, VITAMIN E, SELENIUM, AND CAROTENOIDS

Presenter: Susan Taylor Mayne

Overview

The DRI Antioxidant Report (IOM, 2000b) contains Estimated Average Requirements (EARs), Recommended Dietary Allowances (RDAs), and Tolerable Upper Intake Levels (ULs) for vitamin C, vita-

[1]This chapter is based on a transcript and slides covering the session. Dr. Mayne acknowledged contributions of fellow panelists Raymond Burke and Maret Traber.

min E, and selenium for each life-stage group above age 12 months. In each case, criteria were based on a specific function and not on the prevention of chronic disease. The report also addresses beta-carotene and the carotenoids; but no EARs, RDAs, or ULs were established for any of those substances.

Selenium

Progress Made

Considerable research has been conducted on selenium in the past 6 years. In basic science, for example, 25 genes have been identified that code for selenoproteins. Characterization of these genes is now in progress and is expected to yield useful functional information and clarification of biochemical mechanisms.

Selenoprotein P is now considered a highly promising biomarker for selenium status. It could be considered along with selenium-dependent glutathione peroxidase (the current functional indicator) by a future DRI panel.

Disease prevention was and continues to be a particular area of interest related to the antioxidant nutrients. The ongoing Selenium and Vitamin E Chemoprevention Trial (SELECT), a very large cancer prevention clinical trial involving 35,000 men, will provide much needed clinical data on possible roles of selenium in disease prevention and on adverse effects that may occur with selenium supplementation. The basis for SELECT comes from the Selenium Skin Cancer Prevention Trial (Clark et al., 1996), which studied skin cancer prevention resulting from 4.5 years of supplementation with 200 µg/day of selenium in the form of selenium-enriched yeast. No reduction in second skin cancers occurred; but, unexpectedly, fewer cancers of the prostate, lung, and colorectum were noted in the group that received selenium supplements. The SELECT trial is designed to try to replicate this provocative finding. Figure 5-1 depicts the SELECT study design.

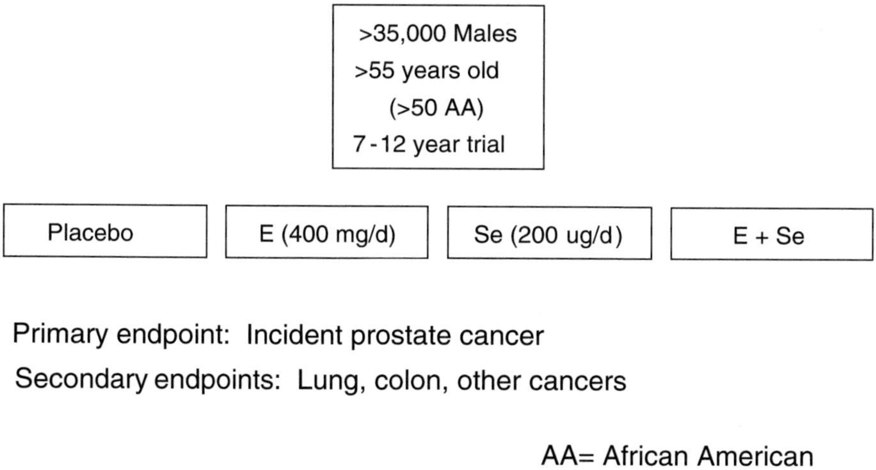

FIGURE 5-1 Overview of Selenium and Vitamin E Chemoprevention Trial (SELECT).

A subgroup analysis of the Nutritional Prevention of Cancer Trial (Duffield-Lillico et al., 2002) addressed efficacy of the selenium supplementation as a function of baseline selenium status. Although the investigators found reductions in incident cancer among subjects in the first and second tertiles of selenium intake at entry (both of which represented low selenium intakes because participants for this study were recruited from low-selenium regions of the United States), there was a 20 percent increase in the risk of total cancer among subjects in the highest tertile of selenium intake. This finding of greater efficacy in persons with lower nutrient status at baseline is supportive of results of some other antioxidant nutrient trials, indicating that baseline nutrient status may be important in determining the efficacy of supplementation with that nutrient.

Although SELECT will provide a wealth of data, a future DRI panel will face challenges in interpreting the results if no benefits are observed. Concerns have been raised about the dose of vitamin E (higher than that used in the Alpha-Tocopherol Beta-Carotene (ATBC) Trial; see further discussion), the form of selenium being used, the timing and duration of the intervention, and lifestyle factors and baseline nutritional status that may modify the effects.

Questions for Future Research

Dr. Mayne raised the following questions for future research concerning selenium:

- Could selenoprotein P be used as the basis for setting the EAR and RDA for selenium?
- What health risks are associated with marginal selenium intake?
- Does supplemental selenium benefit only those with inadequate status?
- What mechanisms are responsible for selenium's health effects? Evidence indicates that there are many possible mechanisms in addition to antioxidant function.

A persistent research gap that applies to all the antioxidant nutrients concerns the nutrient needs of children. Little or no data are available on the nutrient requirements of children or infants.

Vitamin E

Despite the considerable interest in roles of vitamin E in the prevention of chronic disease, the DRI panel on antioxidants determined that the research base was insufficient to allow the use of a chronic disease end point as a functional indicator for setting the EAR and RDA for vitamin E. Instead, the functional indicator selected for those DRI values was the prevention of hydrogen peroxide-induced hemolysis.

Progress Made

Over the past few years, much research attention has been given to vitamin E with regard to basic science progress (ongoing stable isotope studies, for example, will greatly illuminate understanding of metabolism and kinetics for vitamin E), chronic disease studies (especially coronary heart disease prevention studies in high-risk populations), and vitamin E supplementation trials for cancer prevention (primarily among high-risk populations).

The most promising data to come out of the large clinical trials on vitamin E is the possibility of a protective effect of vitamin E against prostate cancer (Virtamo et al., 2003). An unexpected 30 percent reduction in prostate cancer incidence occurred in the ATBC Trial, a lung cancer prevention trial conducted in Finland. In this trial, smokers were randomized to receive vitamin E (50 mg/day) or placebo. Since this was a lung cancer prevention trial rather than a prostate cancer prevention trial and all the subjects in the trial were smoking at entry, questions remain: Is vitamin E protective against prostate cancer? Is the effect limited to smokers only?

Additional evidence suggests that vitamin E may reduce the risk of prostate cancer in smokers only. An observational cohort study (Chan et al., 1999) found that vitamin E supplement use was not related to overall prostate cancer risk. However, among the current smokers or recent quitters in the study, an inverse association was suggested, particularly for metastatic or fatal prostate cancer. The relative risk was 0.44, which was nearly statistically significant. Similarly, in the Prostate, Lung, Colorectal and Ovarian (PLCO) Cancer Screening Trial, supplemental vitamin E was not associated with the overall risk of prostate cancer. With both higher dose and longer duration of vitamin E supplementation, however, a statistically significant decrease in the risk of advanced prostate cancer was observed among current and recent smokers (Kirsh et al., 2006).

Continuing Research Gaps

A continuing research gap relates to the limited information about vitamin E in food composition databases. Data still are not widely available on the alpha-tocopherol, gamma-tocopherol, and delta-tocopherol contents of foods. Moreover, evidence is needed on the biological activity of various vitamin E forms in humans.

Dr. Mayne raised a new question in terms of research challenges; namely, When conducting prevention trials, is it more informative to base the research design on unexpected results from previous trials or to base them on findings from observational epidemiology? SELECT will provide data pertinent to this question.

Beta-Carotene and the Carotenoids

The panel for the DRI Antioxidant Report considered a number of possible functional indicators for beta-carotene and the carotenoids: vitamin A equivalency, markers of antioxidant activity, modulation of gap junctional communication, immune functions, and relationship to chronic diseases such as cancer, coronary heart disease, macular degeneration, and cataract formation. Vitamin A equivalency was addressed by the DRI panel on micronutrients.

Progress Made

Uneven progress has been made. Functional indicators such as gap junctional communication, immune modulation, and antioxidant markers still remain unvalidated as being predictive of a disease outcome. However, dermal carotenoid concentration, measured using noninvasive techniques, is a possible new status indicator.

Although some prevention trial results were available to the panel before publication of the DRI Antioxidants Report in 2000, more recent analyses have identified subgroups that apparently benefit and subgroups that are harmed by supplementation. For example, one of the trials (Baron et al., 2003) found that beta-carotene significantly reduced the risk of colorectal adenoma recurrence in nonsmokers and nondrinkers, and significantly increased it in smokers and drinkers. The Supplémentation en Vitamines et Minéraux Antioxydants (SUVIMAX) trial of many different nutrients, including antioxidant nutrients, found that men benefited and women did not with regard to cancer incidence (the primary outcome studied).

Considerable progress has been made in research related to macular degeneration. The Age-Related Eye Disease Study (AREDS), a randomized clinical trial using antioxidant nutrients and zinc, found that this nutrient combination significantly reduced the risk of advanced macular degeneration among persons who already had some macular changes (Age-Related Eye Disease Study Research Group, 2001). AREDS II will be the first large controlled trial of supplemental lutein and zeaxanthin—carotenoids—for which very little human supplementation data are available. The trial also will include testing of intake of long-chain omega-3 fatty acids.

Critically needed methodologic work has been conducted on the measurement of macular pigment, a possible new status indicator. The new methods (heterochromatic flicker photometry and Raman spectroscopy) have been used in studies that look at determinants (e.g., diet, genetics, and adiposity) of macular pigment. The predictive ability of macular pigment for future disease risk is still unknown—a causal link has not yet been established.

Continuing Research Gaps

Continuing research gaps include the following:

- The dose-dependence of carotenoid effects on health
- Effects of polymorphisms in antioxidant-related or regulated genes on the efficacy of antioxidant nutrients
- The role of oxidative stress in chronic disease
- Predictive value of markers of oxidative stress for clinical end points
- Understanding subgroup effects, especially smoking, which are evident throughout the antioxidant nutrient literature

Development and validation of biomarkers of oxidative stress are still lacking. The prevention of artifact is a big challenge in this work. Moreover, it is necessary to characterize the intra- and intersubject variability of these markers before their use can be explored in population studies.

The DRI Process

DRI Process as Related to Antioxidant Nutrients

Process questions specific to the antioxidant nutrients appear in Box 5-1. With regard to question 1, many nutrients and other food components that have antioxidant function were not addressed by the first panel

BOX 5-1
DRI Process Questions Related to the Antioxidant Nutrients

1. Should antioxidant nutrients be addressed more comprehensively?

2. If a nutrient has beneficial effects at doses much higher than needed for the prevention of deficiency, how should this affect the setting of EARs and RDAs?

3. If vitamin E prevents prostate cancer in smokers but not in nonsmokers, how can this information be incorporated into a DRI process?

4. Should an AI be set for a nutrient that has no known essential functions in humans?

on antioxidants. This applies, for example, to many of the phytochemcals. Question 4 was considered by the first panel on antioxidants, for example, with regard to lycopene.

General Aspects of the Dietary Reference Intake Process

According to Dr. Mayne, a major issue is how to incorporate health promotion into the DRI process. The lack of functional indicators that are associated with the promotion of optimal health limited the ability of the panel on antioxidants to address this. There is a lack of congruity between the public health priority (which is the prevention of chronic diseases) and the current DRI process (which says that a functional indicator is needed to set an EAR or AI). Because of this, all the EARs in the DRI Antioxidant Report are based upon functional indicators, and none are linked to any chronic disease prevention end points. With this in mind, Dr. Mayne raised the question, "Should the concept of a range of nutrient intake be reconsidered, or is there some other method to incorporate information about disease prevention (including subgroup-specific information) into the DRI process? Dr. Mayne invited other speakers to address this issue.

DIETARY REFERENCE INTAKES FOR ANTIOXIDANT NUTRIENTS: GENERAL AND SPECIFIC FRESH PERSPECTIVES

Presenter: John N. Hathcock

The DRI Process

This presentation provided perspectives that relate mainly to the DRI process and included a number of suggestions, which are summarized below.

- Rather than setting the RDA based on a 10 percent or 20 percent coefficient of variation (about two standard deviations higher than the EAR), consider setting it at four standard deviations above the EAR. This would cover the entire population but would not be near the UL. For vitamin E, for example, the values would be as follows:

  - EAR, 12 mg for adult males
  - Current RDA, 15 mg
  - Proposed RDA (EAR plus four standard deviations), 18 mg

- Could risk assessment methodology be used to evaluate the lower end rather than just the upper end of nutrient risk? Figure 5-2 depicts the concept. Dr. Hathcock suggested that examination of the potential advantages and disadvantages of implementing this concept be undertaken by an expert national committee.
- Can the UL concept be expanded to include a value for nutrients for which an adverse effect or a toxicity has not been clearly established, such as vitamin B_{12}? To date, no UL has been set for such nutrients. The lack of a UL might be interpreted in either of two ways: (1) there is no UL because of a lack of adequate data, or (2) there is almost no evidence whatever of toxicity despite ample data. Dr. Hathcock suggested that a value called the Highest Observed Intake in a recent Food and Agriculture Organization and World Health Organization report (FAO/WHO, 2005) (a value that he calls an Observed Safe Level) would be a useful addition.

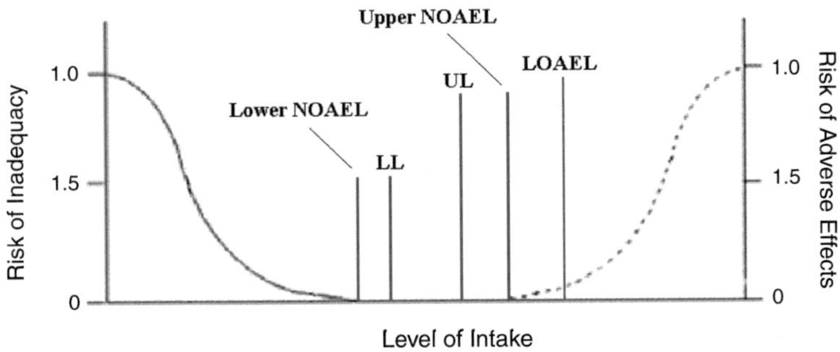

FIGURE 5-2 Hypothetical curve depicting symmetrical risk assessment. NOTE: NOAEL = No Observed Adverse Effect Level, LL = Lower Level, UL = Tolerable Upper Intake Level, LOAEL = Lowest Observed Adverse Effect Level

- Can the process of setting ULs be made more systematic—one that consistently uses a decision tree approach?
- Are separate UL values needed for different forms of a nutrient? Examples include alpha- and gamma-vitamin E and forms of selenium such as selenized yeast, sodium selenide, sodium selenate, and sodium methionine.
- Can risk and benefit curves be prepared for lutein, zeaxanthin, lycopene, and selenium chemical species and modulators for use in setting DRIs?

Other Concerns

In addition, Dr. Hathcock pointed out concerns he had regarding the meta-analysis of high-dosage vitamin E supplementation conducted by Miller and colleagues (2005) (concerns that one of the coauthors rebutted during the discussion period). Dr. Hathcock also raised questions about the advisability of terminating a randomized-controlled trial when clear benefit is seen for a secondary rather than a primary end point (as was the case in the study of selenium supplementation by Clark et al. [1996]). In particular, if a secondary end point is one that automatically has to be retested, is it appropriate to use it as the basis for stopping a study early? In short, Dr. Hathcock stated that there is a need to examine the statistical methods applied to multiple clinical trials and to multiple end points.

DISCUSSION

Discussion centered on concerns related to setting the EAR for vitamin E based on vitamin E concentrations and hydrogen peroxide-induced hemolysis—even though such hemolysis is not a clinical problem. This was the indicator for which data were available; there were insufficient data about other indicators and chronic disease end points that had been considered by the panel. For points raised about how this relates to appropriateness of the model, see the discussion section in Chapter 13.

6

Dietary Reference Intakes for Vitamin A, Vitamin K, Arsenic, Boron, Chromium, Copper, Iodine, Iron, Manganese, Molybdenum, Nickel, Silver, Vanadium, and Zinc[1]

In this session, Robert Russell of Tufts University, former chair of the panel on micronutrients, focused attention on research related to 4 of the 14 disparate nutrients that were covered in the DRI Micronutrients Report (IOM, 2001), namely vitamin A, vitamin K, iron, and zinc.[2] Dr. Janet Hunt of Grand Forks Human Nutrition Research Center, former member of the Subcommittee on Interpretation and Uses of Dietary Reference Intakes, provided research perspectives related to the report.

DISCUSSION OF RESEARCH RECOMMENDATIONS

Presenter: Robert M. Russell

To set the stage for considering research recommendations, this presentation provided background information on Dietary Reference Intakes (DRIs). Then Dr. Russell identified and discussed what he considered to be the four most important research recommendations made in the DRI Micronutrients Report.

---

[1]This chapter is based on a transcript and slides from the workshop.
[2]Dr. Russell's comments incorporate input from a majority of the other micronutrient panel members.

Background Information

The background information provided here is intended to illustrate the major knowledge gaps that have posed challenges for setting DRIs for the micronutrients covered in the DRI Micronutrients Report. The Estimated Average Requirements (EARs) for vitamin A, iron, and zinc were all based on factorial considerations including percent absorption, bioavailability, excretion, turnover, and utilization of the nutrient. The panel had considered using indicators for setting the EARs for these nutrients. Examples of indicators the panel considered when setting the EAR for vitamin A include

- immune function,
- conjunctival impression cytology,
- relative dose–response and modified relative dose–response,
- isotope dilution,
- serum/plasma retinol concentration, and
- dark adaptation.

The first three indicators were not selected either because most of the work was done in animals or because the observations were made in developing countries where the total nutritional profiles were uncertain. Insufficient data were available on isotope dilution studies to obtain a good prediction of body stores of vitamin A. Neither serum nor plasma retinol concentrations could be used because retinol is under homeostatic control.

By pooling data from four studies on dark adaptation, encompassing 13 individuals, the EAR would have been set at 300 retinol activity equivalents (RAEs), Because the coefficient of variation was 40 percent, however, it was judged that the Recommended Dietary Allowance (RDA) could not be established using dark adaptation (the preferred indicator). Thus, the factorial method rather than dark adaptation was used to set the EAR. Doing this resulted in an EAR that was about twice as high—625 RAE/day.

For vitamin K, an Adequate Intake (AI) was set rather than an EAR. This decision was a result of two factors: lack of dose–response data and some uncertainty about the physiologic relevancy of carboxylated osteocalcin as an indicator for vitamin K status.

Four Key Research Recommendations

Dr. Russell identified four research recommendations in the DRI Micronutrients Report that he viewed as of highest priority. These recommendations appear below. These four research recommendations cut across many of the nutrients and remain major research gaps.

1. Identification of new functional and biochemical end points that indicate sufficient and insufficient body stores (vitamin A, vitamin K, iron, chromium)
2. Identification of new functional and biochemical end points that indicate nutrient toxicity (iron and oxidative status, iron content of ferritin, hepcidin, vitamin A and bone toxicity, zinc and immune function)
3. The identification and (quantified) effects of interactions between micronutrients and other food components: calcium and zinc, zinc and phytate
4. Determination of the effects of age, sex, race, pregnancy, and lactation on nutrient utilization and turnover: vitamin A, vitamin K, zinc

Status of These Research Needs

The Identification of New Functional and Biochemical End Points

As an example of the first recommendation, studies are needed of the relationship between early childhood iron deficiency and cognitive function with an eye toward identifying the best indicators of risk. Some progress has been made on vitamin K, and studies are underway. For example, three clinical intervention trials are investigating the specific role of phylloquinone in bone in postmenopausal women. At least one is addressing the beneficial effects of pharmacologic dosing of menaquinone 4 in the treatment of osteoporosis. (Menaquinone 4 has been used to treat osteoporosis for more than 10 years in Japan, with reported benefits [Cockayne et al., 2006].) These three intervention studies should provide useful information about the physiologic significance of undercarboxylated osteocalcin and could be helpful in providing data useful for establishing EARs.

New studies suggest roles for vitamin K in coronary artery disease and in brain function, and these topics warrant further research. For example, strong animal data support a role for vitamin K-dependent proteins as an inhibitor of calcification. In particular, mice lacking the gene coding for matrix Gla protein show calcification of their arteries that leads to hemorrhagic death due to vessel rupture. As another example, animal studies of neurodegeneration hold promise and need to be expanded. In addition, parallel human studies are needed to examine links of neuropsychological outcome measures or other measures of cognitive function with vitamin K status. Because high intakes of vitamin K are associated with high-quality diets, prospective intervention trials using the isolated vitamin will be needed to distinguish the action of vitamin K from that of other nutrients, such as folate.

End Points that Indicate Nutrient Toxicity

A number of functional and biochemical end points that indicate nutrient toxicity offer promising avenues of research:

- Iron and oxidative status, iron content of ferritin, and hepcidin
- The relationship between iron status, serum ferritin, and the metabolic syndrome and the putative risk for cardiovascular diseases related to oxidative damage
- The examination of which systems become dysfunctional with excess zinc, considering the immune system as a prime target of investigation
- The relationship of vitamin A intake with bone demineralization—Feskanich and coworkers (2002) provide evidence that this adverse effect occurs at intakes that are close to the RDA, but some inconsistent findings also have been reported

Interactions

Of particular interest are studies of interactions between calcium and zinc and between zinc and phytate. Related is study of the quantity of endogenous zinc excreted by the intestine versus the quantity absorbed (i.e., studies on human zinc homeostasis) at various intake levels.

Effects of Age, Sex, Race, and Physiological Status on Nutrient Utilization

The DRI values set for children (by the use of extrapolation) merit attention. Table 6-1, which covers vitamin A values, illustrates this point.

One can see that the Tolerable Upper Intake Levels (ULs) for the younger children equal the RDAs for adolescents—a situation that calls for closer examination. Similarly for the younger children, the UL for zinc is very close to the RDA; and it could be easy for young children to exceed the UL for zinc.

The investigation of lactating women's iodine requirements is another topic still in need of research.

TABLE 6-1 Selected Dietary Reference Intake Values for Vitamin A and the Criteria Used to Set Them, by Life Stage

Life Stage	Criterion	EAR	RDA	AI	UL
		←μg of vitamin A/day→			
0–6 months	Human milk content			400	
7–12 months	Extrapolated from 0–6 months			500	
1–2 years	Extrapolated from adults	210	300		600
4–8 years	Extrapolated from adults	275	400		900
9–13 years, M	Extrapolated from adults	445	600		
9–13 years, F	Extrapolated from adults	420	600		
14–18 years, M	Extrapolated from adults	630	900		
14–18 years, F	Extrapolated from adults	485	700		
> 18 years, M	Adequate body stores	625	900		
> 18 years, F	Adequate body stores	500	700		

M = Male; F = Female; EAR = Estimated Average Requirement; RDA = Recommended Dietary Allowance; AI = Adequate Intake; UL = Tolerable Upper Intake Level.

SOURCE: IOM (2001).

Research Gaps for Which New Data Are Available

More data are available now to address a number of research questions identified by the panel on micronutrients, including the following:

- The effect of vitamin A status on plant carotene conversion. The lower the vitamin A nutriture, the better humans break down and utilize the plant carotene (Ribaya-Mercado et al., 2000).
- The vitamin A activity of different plant foods (Haskell et al., 2004; Tang et al., 1999; 2005). For example, the conversion ratio of beta-carotene to vitamin A would be 21 μg to 1 μg for spinach and 15 to 1 for carrots. Research is still needed on how this conversion is affected when the plant food is eaten as a part of a whole meal.
- The vitamin A content of foods
- Classifications of iron-loading syndromes with identification of the central role of hepcidin, which is a down-regulator of iron transport. There is great hope that hepcidin could be used in setting an EAR and/or in considering iron overload.

Potential New Research Questions

Dr. Russell posed a set of topics for investigation that have arisen since the writing of the DRI Micronutrients Report:

- Vitamin A and gene expression profiles, especially gene expressions that control certain functions
- The bioavailability and metabolism of menaquinones and the roles of menaquinones and phyloquinones in sphingolipid metabolism. Animal data published since the DRI Micronutrients Report completion points to roles for vitamin K in the form of menaquinone for brain function: it stimulates sphingolipid synthesis and improves cognition.
- The relationship between iron status and infections, such as human immunodeficiency virus (HIV) and tuberculosis
- Food-specific bioavailability questions, such as the bioavailability of iron or beta-carotene in cereal and legume crops produced by varietal selection or genetic engineering to improve iron or vitamin A nutrition

- Biomarkers of zinc status, primarily genomic or proteomic, to correlate with functional outcomes such as immunity. For example, a gene product derived from zinc-influenced systems (such as zinc transporter proteins) might serve as a biomarker.

Status of Research on Chromium, Copper, and Ultra-Trace Minerals

No substantial progress has been made on the bioavailability and turnover of chromium, copper, or the ultra-trace minerals (arsenic, boron, manganese, molybdenum, nickel, silicon, and vanadium). Furthermore, no substantial data have been published to date on physiologic and psychologic functional consequences of deficiencies of these minerals. A research question might be, "What is the effect of boron deficiency in bone health?"

Summary

In summary, for vitamin K, much progress has occurred and more is expected over the next several years—probably enough on which to base an EAR. For vitamin A, there has been substantial progress as well. Despite good progress for iron, much remains to be done, especially regarding hepcidin as a marker of iron status. For the other minerals, much work still needs to be done.

RESEARCH PERSPECTIVES

Presenter: Janet R. Hunt

The DRI process can be related to the circular process of assessment, planning, implementation, and evaluation (Figure 6-1). Following the steps in Figure 6-1 can help to identify research needs.

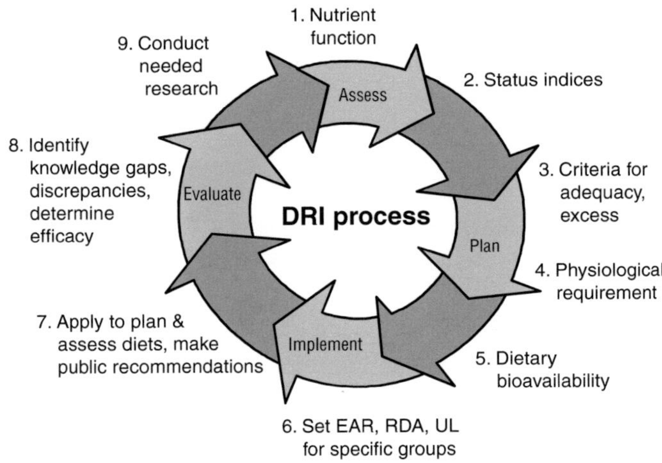

FIGURE 6-1 Dietary Reference Intakes process in relation to the circular assessment, planning, implementation, and evaluation process.

Steps 1 and 2: Nutrient Function and Status Indicators

There is a need to identify the functional roles related to good health for the micronutrients. Even though zinc is widely known for its importance for immune function and for wound healing, it is not yet possible to identify a specific immune function, chemical, or indicator that can be used to indicate adequate zinc intake.

Sensitive status indices are lacking for the micronutrients covered in the DRI Micronutrients Report, with the possible exceptions of vitamin A, iron, and iodine. For example, beyond the prevention of anemia and having adequate levels of transferrin saturation, there currently is no clear-cut point for measurement indicators of iron stores. It is notable that since the DRI Micronutrients Report was completed, Cook and colleagues (2003) have developed a measure of body iron stores by using an algorithm based on the ratio of serum transferrin receptor (TfR) and serum ferritin. However, the measure does not provide a clear-cut point for adequacy. In intervention studies in developing countries, this algorithm using TfR and serum ferritin has been very sensitive. In contrast to using hemoglobin as an end point, this algorithm-based method of measuring body iron stores can be used in intervention studies to reduce the number of subjects and shorten the observation time. However, there is a strong need for standardization of the measurement of TfR between different commercial assays.

As Dr. Russell indicated, hepcidin is a very promising general indicator of iron status—namely, as a regulator of iron absorption in the body (Nemeth and Ganz, 2006). However, most hepcidin data have been limited to genetic expression in animals, and the measurement of hepcidin peptide in serum poses challenges. Research is needed to develop the methodology and to apply hepcidin to the assessment of iron status in humans (Hadley et al., 2006). Dr. Hunt also agreed that status indices related to iron and cognition are needed, especially to address concerns about childhood iron deficiency and its impact on cognition and possibly mood and affect.

Further research on zinc transport proteins (Liuzzi and Cousins, 2004) may provide a more specific indicator of nutritional adequacy that could contribute to setting the EAR for zinc. This area of research requires more animal as well as human studies to identify sensitive and specific indicators.

The few functional indices available do not provide evidence that the use of mineral supplements will affect performance, as concluded in a recent review of mineral requirements for military personnel (IOM, 2006b); but the identification of functional indices continues to be an area of research that would support the development of DRIs.

Steps 3 and 4: Criteria and Physiological Requirement

The ability to set criteria for adequacy and excess is limited when the criteria cannot be based on function. This is the case, for example, when one must rely on factorial estimations of nutrient requirements.

Basing an EAR or AI on factorial estimations of the requirement relies largely on the use of data from balance studies and the replacement of estimated daily excretion. To the extent that such studies must servc as the basis of requirements, Dr. Hunt supports the report's recommendations for research methods that call for balance studies that (1) are sufficiently long to reach a new steady state, and (2) are designed so that the intakes bracket the requirements. When making factorial estimations, an additional consideration is the handling of nutrient loss through sweat. Specific situations of heat and humidity affect sweat losses of nutrients, but they are very difficult to measure accurately, and data are lacking regarding how adaptation affects such losses (IOM, 2006b).

Step 5: Dietary Bioavailability

Accounting for the Bioavailability of Iron

The bioavailability of iron merits special attention as related to the EAR and RDA. In particular, the EAR for iron was based on an estimated 18 percent iron bioavailability from a typical North American dietary intake. However, a diet consistent with the recently released *Dietary Guidelines for Americans 2005* (DHHS/USDA, 2005) may reduce the bioavailability of iron to approximately 11 percent, (Hunt, unpublished calculation). This estimate is based on the much higher fiber content recommended by *Dietary Guidelines for Americans 2005* (which is consistent with the AI for dietary fiber). An 11 percent bioavailability suggests that the dietary iron requirement would be 60 percent larger than if the bioavailability were 18 percent. Given that the same amount of iron consumed can result in vastly different amounts of iron absorbed, perhaps iron recommendations need to incorporate bioavailability considerations and suggestions for improving iron bioavailability rather than be limited to the amount of iron to be consumed.

Progress Made

Since 2002, some progress has been made regarding the bioavailability of both zinc and iron. The International Zinc Nutrition Consultative Group has developed an algorithm that predicts zinc bioavailability from the whole diet (International Zinc Nutrition Consultative Group, 2004). It is based on two factors: the zinc content of the diet and the phytate content of the diet. Recognition has increased that the oral zinc dose or the amount of zinc in a meal affects zinc absorptive efficiency (International Zinc Nutrition Consultative Group, 2004). Work also has progressed on the bioavailability of different forms of zinc, including indication that zinc oxide is bioavailable and could be useful for fortification (Herman et al., 2002; de Romana et al., 2003).

Step 6: Setting EARs, RDAs, and ULs for Specific Groups

Problems posed by the need to extrapolate to set DRIs for children have, in several instances, resulted in setting a UL that is lower than typical intakes of specific age groups. In particular, based on data from the Continuing Survey of Food Intakes by Individuals, substantial percentages of formula-fed infants and of children up to age 8 years have zinc intakes that exceed the UL. Similarly, high percentages of children have iodine intakes that exceed the UL. Reported intakes of vitamin A also commonly exceed the UL for children younger than the age of 4 years.

Step 7: Applying Dietary Reference Intakes in Planning and Assessing Diets

Apparent discrepancies have been discovered when applying the new DRIs to the planning and assessment of diets. For example, discrepancies between intakes and the UL for manganese appear for subgroups of individuals. Typical diets of some groups, such as pregnant women and vegetarians, may not be adequate for iron. Because of lower dietary iron bioavailability, the benefit of iron supplementation of vegetarian diets is unclear.

Steps 8 and 9: Identifying Knowledge Gaps and Discrepancies and Conducting Needed Research

A number of knowledge gaps and discrepancies were identified above. In addition, knowledge of the usefulness of different supplemental forms of iron, including different elemental iron powders and chelated forms of iron, has increased (Hurrell et al., 2002; Swain et al., 2003; Hoppe et al., 2003; Zimmerman et al., 2005). In Vietnamese and Chinese studies, sodium iron ethylendiaminetetra-acetic acid (EDTA) has been shown to be very effective in addressing iron deficiency anemia (Chen et al., 2005; Van Thuy et al., 2005).

For elements such as boron, there is potential that further research information, probably beginning with animal models, might lead to inclusion as a nutrient. Boron is demonstrated to be essential for most of the plant world (Devirian and Volpe, 2003).

DISCUSSION

Comments and questions following this presentation were of a general nature and are summarized in Chapter 13, "Wrap-up Session."

7

Dietary Reference Intakes for Energy, Carbohydrate, Fiber, Fat, Fatty Acids, Cholesterol, Protein, and Amino Acids[1]

During this session, Joanne Lupton of Texas A&M University, former chair of the panel on macronutrients, discussed selected research recommendations covering the five types of nutrients in the Dietary Reference Intakes (DRI) Macronutrients Report (IOM, 2002/2005). Harold Kohl of the Centers for Disease Control and Prevention (CDC) addressed research recommendations pertaining to physical activity, and Joanne Slavin of the University of Minnesota, St. Paul, provided perspectives on research recommendations pertaining to fiber.

DISCUSSION OF RESEARCH RECOMMENDATIONS

Presenter: Joanne R. Lupton

This presentation on the knowledge gaps and research gaps from the DRI Macronutrients Report (IOM, 2002/2005) covered specific research recommendations if they met one or more of the following criteria:

- The research has a direct effect on either changing a current DRI value or the criteria upon which that value is established. This could include providing sufficient data to move from an Adequate Intake (AI) to a Recommended Dietary Allowance (RDA), for example.

[1]This chapter is based on a transcript and slides from the workshop.

- The research results could be used in establishing a new DRI value.
- The handling of the topic in the DRI Macronutrients Report generated much discussion within the professional community.
- The research is related to DRI values that were difficult to meet as a part of eating plans that are consistent with the *Dietary Guidelines for Americans 2005* (DHHS/USDA, 2005).

Background information of the derivation of specific Estimated Average Requirements (EARs), RDAs, or AIs is provided to help clarify the continuing research needs.

Carbohydrates

Recommended Dietary Allowance

With regard to carbohydrates, there is much controversy over the RDA of 130 grams of carbohydrate per day and over the recommendation that intake of added sugars be less than 25 percent of calories. In addition, a recommendation to revisit the difference between high-glycemic and low-glycemic diets on diabetes and coronary heart disease needs attention.

The RDA of 130 grams of carbohydrate per day is based on the amount of glucose needed by the brain in a day. That amount of carbohydrate, however, is less than the amount that would be the lower limit of the Acceptable Macronutrient Distribution Range (AMDR). Thus, there is reason to consider basing the RDA for carbohydrate on the overall diet. Notably, the carbohydrate RDA was not used in developing the *Dietary Guidelines for Americans 2005* (DHHS/USDA, 2004, 2005). In this example, the research question might be, What level of carbohydrate intake is commensurate with a healthy diet?

Added Sugars

The recommendation to limit added sugars to no more than 25 percent of calories was derived from a review of all the studies that examined the intake of added sugars and its relationship to micronutrient intake. The cutoff point at which decreased intake of micronutrients appears to become statistically significant is approximately 25 percent of calories coming from added sugars.

Three longitudinal studies that show an increase in weight gain with added sugars from certain sources have been released since 2002 (Berkey et al., 2004; Mrdjenovic and Levitsky, 2003; Phillips et al., 2004). Other studies are in progress. These new data show that over time, in the same group of individuals, weight gain occurs if one consumes added sugars, especially if the sugars are obtained from soft drinks (sodas). Importantly, to develop food patterns that follow the 2005 Dietary Guidelines and meet nutrient needs and energy, most of one's energy must be obtained from the food groups, and very few calories are available to use in the form of added sugars.

Discretionary calories was the name given by the Dietary Guidelines Advisory Committee (DHHS/USDA, 2004) for the difference between energy needs and the energy provided by servings from the food groups to meet nutrient needs. Added sugars fit into the discretionary calories category. Thus, Dr. Lupton suggested considering the new literature and the ongoing studies on added sugars and weight gain, and how many discretionary calories can be consumed without gaining weight.

Glycemic Response

The research on the glycemic response to the diet is advancing to the point where a panel might make specific recommendations. The need now is for clinical intervention trials that compare diets with high glycemic index or load to diets with low glycemic index or load, using appropriate end points, including diabetes, hemoglobin A1c, blood glucose, and blood insulin.

Fiber

An AI was set for total fiber, which includes the fiber from foods (dietary fiber) and the fiber that is synthesized or extracted and added to foods (functional fiber). Decreased risk of coronary heart disease was the end point used. Although the recommendation was based on the totality of fiber and coronary heart disease (CHD) research, the specific numbers for the DRI value were generated from three prospective trials. Dr. Lupton stated that a randomized clinical trial, preferably with three levels of fiber intake and surrogate markers for CHD, would be necessary to move from an AI to an EAR for fiber. Alternatively, a panel might consider changing the clinical end point from decreased risk of CHD to improved bowel health or healthy laxation, for example. Many studies with relevant data have been published, but agreement on the definition of healthy laxation or bowel health would be required.

Considerable concern has been expressed that the AI of 14 grams of fiber per 1,000 calories is too high for children. Thus, a research need is to study the effect of fiber intake, specifically in children.

A pertinent research question is whether a difference in overall health occurs if the fiber in a high-fiber diet is derived mainly from dietary fiber versus functional fiber. Would the end point be the same? To date, nearly all the research papers cover dietary fiber.

Dr. Lupton indicated that each fiber source that is promoted or suggested as a functional fiber needs to be tested for efficacy before it is added to the food supply. In addition, she raised a question about the potential for adverse effects from consuming too high a fiber intake from foods to which functional fiber has been added and whether there is a need for a Tolerable Upper Intake Level (UL) for functional fiber.

Fatty Acids, Fat, and Cholesterol

The report includes AIs for linoleic acid and for alpha-linolenic acid, the two essential fatty acids. Because the research literature was scant, the AI values were based on median intakes in the United States. It probably is important to revisit DRIs for fatty acids, particularly for *n*-3 fatty acids, to consider health promotion rather than deficiency symptoms. Also, considerable research published since 2002 concerning docosahexaenoic acid (DHA) and eicosapentaenoic acid (EPA) merits consideration with regard to setting DRI values for these two fatty acids.

See the DRI Macronutrients Report (IOM, 2002/2005) for reasons why there is currently no UL for saturated fat, trans fat, or cholesterol. According to Dr. Lupton, this lack presents a conundrum that needs to be addressed. She proposed a research recommendation to determine the lowest levels of saturated fat, trans fat, and cholesterol that are consistent with a healthy diet and that may cause a low but acceptable amount of harm.

Amino Acids

Because insufficient data were available on dose–response relationships, no ULs were set for amino acids even though some of them are known to result in toxic effects at high doses. This research gap continues to merit attention.

Energy and Physical Activity

With regard to energy and physical activity, it is notable that the single-most contentious issue in this report is the recommendation for one hour of moderate intensity physical activity per day to maintain normal body mass index. Three major research needs include the following:

1. Expand the doubly labeled water database.
2. Determine the effect of physical activity on overall health and wellness rather than solely on body weight and/or risk of disease.
3. Decide on the place and significance of physical activity in the overall arsenal of efforts to promote public health. These efforts include the DRI process, the Dietary Guidelines for Americans, and food intake surveys.

RESEARCH PRIORITIES: ENERGY AND PHYSICAL ACTIVITY FRESH PERSPECTIVES

Presenter: Harold W. Kohl

This presentation provided background information on physical activity as related to Dietary Guidelines for Americans and then focused on a selection of the many specific research recommendations contained in the DRI Macronutrients Report.

Physical Activity and Dietary Guidelines for Americans

Physical activity was incorporated in the Dietary Guidelines for Americans in 1990 when the role of physical activity for energy balance was first acknowledged. Over the ensuing years, physical activity gained increasing recognition in the guidelines. Most recently, in 2005, a specific recommendation was made that both adults and children should accumulate 60 minutes of daily moderate intensity physical activity in addition to the activities required to maintain a sedentary lifestyle to prevent weight gain and to promote additional health benefits.

Status of Research Recommendations Pertaining to Energy and Physical Activity

The DRI Macronutrients Report (IOM, 2002/2005) contains 30 specific recommendations for energy (13 labeled as major knowledge gaps, 13 as knowledge gaps, and 4 as research methods), and an additional 18 specific recommendations for physical activity (only 4 of which are labeled as major knowledge gaps, 13 as knowledge gaps, and 1 as a research method).

Energy Expenditure and Weight Gain or Loss

Dr. Kohl focused on a few of the research recommendations, with his selections influenced by recent research findings. In particular, he took the position that emerging data now suggest that recommendations for patterns of energy expenditure and physical activity differ for the prevention of weight gain, for weight loss, and for the prevention of weight gain after a substantial weight loss. This information is relevant to children, adults, older adults, and pregnant and lactating women.

Regarding the prevention of weight gain, a key question is, What physical activity and energy expenditure patterns will prevent weight gain and for whom, and how would this interact with dietary intake (including diet composition)? Dr. Kohl considers research recommendation number 271-E[2] (regarding energy requirements of overweight and obese individuals and their relationship to physical activity patterns) to be extremely critical in helping to answer this question. Some data suggest that the patterns for energy requirements for overweight and obese people may be different than those for people who never gain weight or who maintain their weight over time.

---

[2]To find the exact wording of each research recommendation to which an identification code corresponds, see Appendix C.

An understanding is needed of some of the longitudinal aspects of physical activity in preventing weight gain. Dr. Kohl repeatedly emphasized investigation of the form, frequency, intensity, and duration of exercise and physical activity in relation to the successful management of body weight.

With regard to weight loss strategies, why do existing data not support an additional benefit of physical activity (above dietary restriction)?

Methods

Some of the disparate results seen in studies of weight loss and of the prevention of weight gain or weight regain may be methodologically driven. Thus, there is a need for reliable, noninvasive, and clinically appropriate measurements of body composition, cardiovascular function, and fitness. Much more thorough assessments are needed regarding the form, frequency, and intensity and duration of exercise, and on their interactions as related to long-term risk for weight gain. Dr. Kohl considers it absolutely essential to expand the doubly labeled water studies of total energy expenditure, giving attention to the need for prospective data, adequate representation of age groups and ethnic groups, and a randomly selected set of study subjects.

Exercise and Substrate Utilization

Research on the effects of exercise on substrate utilization remains an important recommendation. Moderate intensity physical activity—namely, less than about six metabolic equivalents—preferentially oxidizes lipids and lipoproteins. Once the physical activity becomes vigorous, carbohydrates oxidize. Information is needed, however, on the effect of having the same dose of physical activity in terms of kilocalories but under different conditions. For example, two groups could burn the same number of kilocalories if individuals in one group have moderate intensity physical activity for a specific duration, and those in the other group are vigorously active for a shorter period. How would such an interaction help in understanding the process of weight loss?

Possible New Research Questions

Possible new research questions include the following:

- *By what mechanisms does it appear that formerly obese persons may need 60 to 90 minutes of physical activity daily to maintain weight loss?* Some of the strongest data from randomized trials show that people who have lost a substantial amount of weight (which might be 30, 40, or 50 pounds or some significant percentage of their body weight) have a different energy requirement than do people who have not lost weight or who have lost weight and then regained.
- *What behavioral, environmental, policy, and other factors help people adhere to a physical activity and exercise strategy to help maximize their potential for maintenance of weight loss?* Some data indicate that the people who exercise more frequently and who adhere to their physical activity regimens are more likely to maintain their weight loss. In the physical activity literature, evidence-based strategies have been identified that promote physical activity, both on the individual and on the environmental level. Thus, Dr. Kohl recommended that more attention be given to understanding factors influencing these behaviors.
- *To what extent do differences in body composition and fat-free mass need to be considered in studies—rather than just considering differences in body mass index?*

Figure 7-1 illustrates several different conceptual relationships between physical activity and risk of selected diseases. Notably, consistent inverse associations exist between physical activity and the disease outcomes presented. Moreover, higher amounts of physical activity are associated with a continuing lower risk of disease outcome, but at an increasingly diminishing level. The major exception may be musculoskeletal injury. All these relationships together suggest that there are different kinds of associations of physical activity that go beyond weight, body fat, and obesity. In fact, it may be advisable to consider developing a process for physical activity recommendations that would parallel the process for the Dietary Guidelines, with updating of the recommendations perhaps every 5 years.

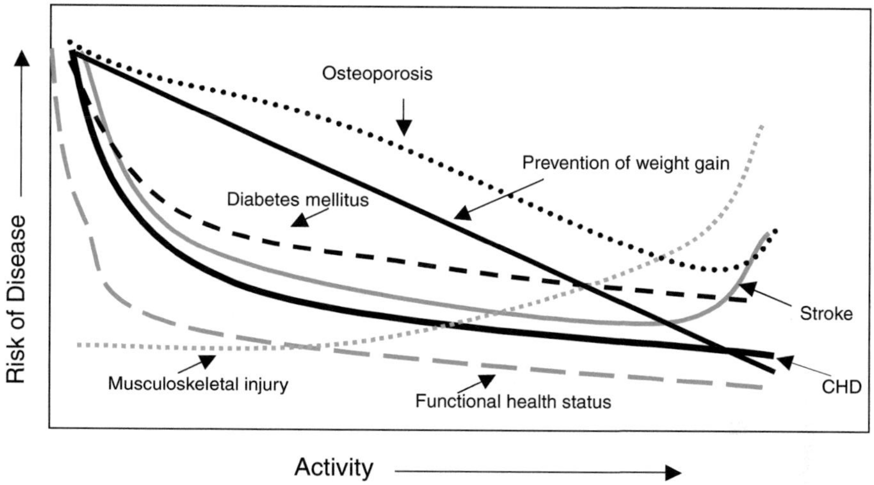

FIGURE 7-1 Risk curves with increasing physical activity, by disease or condition.
NOTE: CHD = coronary heart disease.

FIBER RESEARCH UPDATE

Presenter: Joanne L. Slavin

This presentation began with a very brief history of the evolution of dietary fiber, as illustrated by Figure 7-2, and the periodic "rediscovery" of fiber—culminating with the issuance of fiber definitions and AIs for fiber by the Institute of Medicine (IOM, 2002/2005). Additional topics included considerations for setting DRI values for fiber, research progress, and research questions that merit more attention.

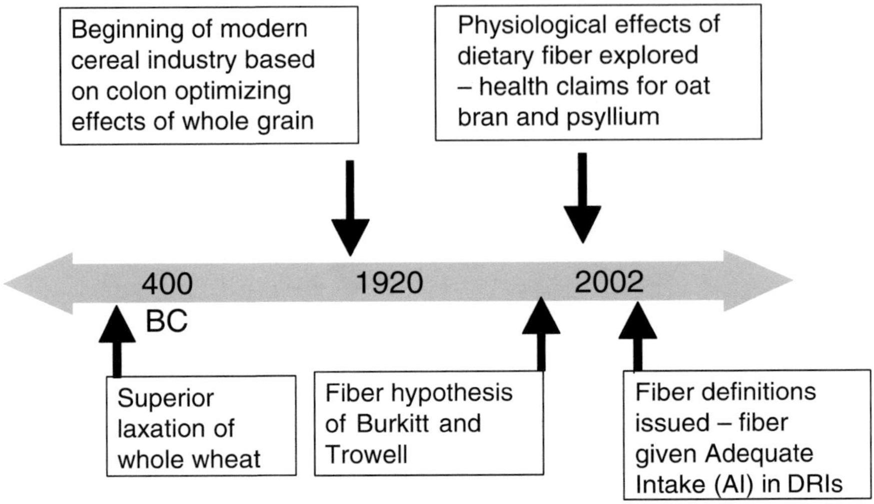

FIGURE 7-2 Highlights of the evolution of attention to dietary fiber, 400 BC–AD 2002.

Considerations for Setting DRI Values for Fiber

Unlike the case for most other nutrients, the recommended intake of fiber was based on protection against disease, not another functional end point. Dr. Slavin agreed with Dr. Lupton that applying the adult AI for fiber (14 g/1,000 kcal) to set the AI for children leads to a higher AI than needed. The AIs for children are much higher than earlier recommendations (e.g., the recommended number of grams of fiber per day equals five plus the child's age); such recommendations were made by other expert groups and were based mainly on intakes. Applying the same ratio (14 g of fiber/1,000 kcal) to elderly adults results in a lower absolute AI than for younger adults. This appears inconsistent considering older persons' concerns about getting enough fiber. The AIs for children and the elderly are based on a calorie conversion factor, not on empirical data. In fact, since fiber was just designated as a nutrient, less relevant human research has been conducted than is the case for some of the other nutrients. In contrast, much useful research related to pet animals and pigs may be available.

Because fiber is nondigestible, it seems obvious that information about fecal material could be used as an indicator in setting DRIs for fiber, and the DRI macronutrients panel investigated that possibility. However, inconsistencies arise when relating fiber intake to either stool output or to a marker in the stool. In part, this is due to the many factors in addition to fiber intake that affect laxation including

- stress,
- exercise (Oettle, 1991),
- smoking,
- coffee drinking,
- drugs (Lembo and Camilleri, 2003),
- personality (Tucker et al., 1981), and
- type of fiber (per gram of fiber fed, wheat produces a greater weight of stool than do oats, and oats produce a greater weight of stool than does pectin [Cummings, 1993]; most types of fiber have not been studied).

The definition of normal laxation—from three or more stools per week to three or fewer stools per day—covers a wide range. Moreover, definitions related to laxation have some inconsistencies. For example, stool weight greater than 200 g/day has been clinically defined as diarrhea (Fine and Schiller, 1999), but many vegetarians have stool weights of 300 g/day or more.

Research on laxation presents some obvious problems. Collecting fecal samples is not practical in epidemiological studies. Moreover, there is no accepted standard with regard to stool weight, stool chemistry, microflora (preferred methods and desirability of different organisms), stool frequency (promising because it is easy data to collect), or quality of life (a measure used in irritable bowel syndrome trials).

Research Progress

The DRI Macronutrients Report contains 12 research recommendations pertaining to fiber—all of which Dr. Slavin rated as highly important, and most of which involved some collection of fecal samples. Because essentially no investigators are collecting fecal samples, little progress has occurred.

Research progress has been made, however, with regard to the relationship of dietary fiber and C-reactive protein (CRP) concentrations. Ajani et al. (2004), using data from the 1999–2000 National Health and

Nutrition Examination Survey, reported that dietary fiber intake is inversely associated with serum CRP. The odds ratio for increased CRP was 0.49 for the highest quintile of fiber intake compared with the lowest. In addition, Ma and colleagues (2006) conducted a longitudinal study of 529 subjects and reported that dietary fiber intake is protective against high CRP.

Despite the strong and consistent evidence that higher levels of fiber intake are protective against CHD, it remains unclear why the data are so strong. It may be in part because of serum cholesterol lowering, but also perhaps because of lower CRP.

Research Questions That Merit More Attention

Some big questions regarding dietary fiber and functional fiber merit more attention. What measurements should be recommended for investigating effects of feeding functional fibers? Are the most important parameters effects on blood cholesterol, CRP, microflora, stool weight, or other? What studies would provide a sound basis for setting fiber recommendations for children, adolescents, and older people? Dr. Slavin considers it important to revise the AI for children and adolescents.

Most of the 12 research recommendations call for basic information, such as feeding dose amounts of fibers and measuring stool weight. Dr. Slavin pointed out that accomplishing these studies will take dedicated research funding because such research would not be funded in the competitive research arena. If food or fiber companies want to know that the fiber has a specific health effect, they might be interested in conducting research that provides information that a regulatory agency will request in the future.

DISCUSSION

Questions and comments during the discussion period focused mainly on (1) the relationship of discretionary calories to the RDA and to energy expenditure, and (2) carbohydrate recommendations.

Discretionary Calories

Discussants disagreed about the value of the concept of discretionary calories and noted that the concept is difficult to communicate effectively. Dr. Murphy clarified that the RDA is about 120 percent of the EAR, not the much higher amounts stated during the discussion. Several discussants pointed out that physical activity is the factor that has the biggest impact on discretionary calories. Dr. Kohl mentioned Jean Meyer's studies in the 1950s that suggested a physical activity threshold below which energy regulation may be impaired, and Dr. Dwyer encouraged replication of those studies.

Carbohydrate Recommendations

Dr. Bier noted the essentiality of glucose for the brain and suggested that the problem is not the carbohydrate RDA but a communication issue. Dr. Lupton agreed that carbohydrate recommendations led to misunderstandings, especially with regard to the recommendation not to exceed an added sugars intake of 25 percent of energy intake.

8

Dietary Reference Intakes for Water, Potassium, Sodium, Chloride, and Sulfate[1]

RESEARCH RECOMMENDATIONS AND OTHER ISSUES

Presenter: Lawrence J. Appel

In this session, Lawrence J. Appel of Johns Hopkins University, who chaired the panel on Dietary Reference Intakes (DRIs) for electrolytes and water, presented a brief overview of the DRIs for sodium, potassium, water, and sulfate; covered research recommendations specific to those nutrients; and addressed some related issues concerning the DRI taxonomy, evidence-based medicine and nutrition policy, and general research. The DRI Electrolytes and Water Report (IOM, 2005) is the most recently published DRI report.

Overview

The DRI Electrolytes and Water Report provides no Estimated Average Requirements (EARs) or Recommended Dietary Allowances (RDAs). Instead, it gives Adequate Intakes (AIs) for water, sodium, and potassium, but no AI value for sulfate. A Tolerable Upper Intake Level (UL) was set for sodium but for none of the other nutrients. This background information is provided to help highlight major knowledge gaps.

---

[1]This chapter is based on a transcript and slides from the workshop.

Rationales for Adequate Intakes

The rationales for the AIs vary by nutrient and are summarized in Box 8-1.

Water For water, the focus primarily was on dehydration as an end point, and serum or plasma osmolality was the indicator used. Examining data on water intake and osmolality from the Third National Health and Nutrition Examination Survey, no evidence of dehydration was found in the general population, even at the first decile of water intake. Serum osmolality basically was identical across the reported intakes. Thus the median water intake was used to set the AI, which is consistent with the definition of AI.

Sodium For sodium, "nutrient adequacy" refers to the sodium intake level at which one could consume a diet that basically meets all the recommended dietary intakes for other nutrients. Of several hypothesized adverse effects of *inadequate* sodium intake, only nutrient inadequacy and volume depletion in the setting of acute thermal stress were considered to be sufficiently well documented to use in setting the AI.

Potassium A controlled feeding study (Morris et al., 1999) was one of several pieces of data that contributed to the basis for the AI of 1,500 mg (120 millimoles) of potassium per day. The investigators fed different

BOX 8-1
Rationale for Adequate Intake, by Nutrient

Nutrient	Rationale
Water	• Median observed in NHANES III for age group
Sodium	• Nutrient adequacy • Buffer in the setting of excess sodium loss during acute sweat losses
Potassium	• Lower blood pressure • Reduce salt sensitivity • Reduce risk of kidney stones • Decrease bone loss

NHANES III = Third National Health and Nutrition Examination Survey

amounts of potassium and then challenged the subjects with salt to see what percentage of individuals experienced a blood pressure increase that was greater than 3 mm Hg. Morris and colleagues reported a steady reduction in salt sensitivity with increasing intakes of potassium. A question that remains is whether it is potassium or some concomitant nutrient (specifically one or more anions) that might be contributing to the protective effect.

Rationale for Tolerable Upper Intake Level for Sodium

In terms of the adverse effects of excess sodium intake, several potential outcomes were considered, but increased blood pressure was the adverse effect used as the basis for setting the UL.

Current Status of Research Recommendations

Because the report was released in 2004, one cannot expect a large amount of progress in filling research gaps. For the nutrients covered in the DRI Electrolytes and Water Report, data were lacking that would be useful in setting EARs or AIs for infants, children, pregnant women, and the elderly—as was the case for most other nutrients. A summary of the current status of research recommendations on sodium and potassium, water, and sulfate follows.

Sodium and Potassium

- With regard to the development of effective public health strategies to achieve and sustain reduced sodium intake and to increase potassium intakes in the general population, activities are underway at the National Heart, Lung, and Blood Institute of the National Institutes of Health, in the New York City Health Department, and in Great Britain.
- Progress regarding the recommendation to develop alternative processing technologies to reduce sodium content of foods is uncertain because much of the relevant information is proprietary.
- An investigator-initiated proposal has been developed for a large-scale trial to test the efficacy of increased potassium intake,

alone and in combination with reduced sodium intake, on prevention of stroke; however, funding for such work is difficult to obtain.

- A few pilot studies are under way to test the main and interactive effects of sodium and potassium intake on bone mineral density and, if possible, bone fractures.
- Only one trial of potassium intake on kidney stones has been conducted, and that study addresses recurrent stones rather than the risk of kidney stones.
- A creative method is being used to assess—without a major new effort—the impact of sodium reduction on clinical cardiovascular events. (The research recommendation called for a formal assessment of the feasibility of a large-scale, long-term clinical trial designed for this purpose.) In particular, a publication is in process that has followed long-term (10 to 15 years) participants who were enrolled in two trials of hypertension prevention. Together, these two trials have documented about a 20 percent reduction in the risk of cardiovascular events.

One interesting line of research relates to the recommendation to conduct randomized trials to compare the effects of different potassium salts on blood pressure and other outcomes at different levels of sodium intake. The effects of anions had been specified as of low priority for the panel. Research by He (2005) indicates that potassium citrate and potassium chloride had similar effects on blood pressure. For bone, in contrast, the anion may have considerable effect.

Dr. Appel views the recommendation to conduct trials that assess the effects of high potassium intake on serum potassium levels and blood pressure in the setting of early stages of kidney disease to be very important from a public health perspective. Although potassium is beneficial in the majority of the population (those with normal kidney function), potassium starts to be harmful as soon as some evidence of kidney dysfunction develops. Given that several million people in the United States alone have chronic kidney disease, it appears very important to determine the point at which a change from benefit to harm occurs. The problem is further exacerbated because angiotensin-converting enzyme inhibitors (medications that commonly are used in the setting of renal disease) tend to increase serum potassium concentration. Such research, however, would involve some substantive methodological challenges.

Water

Dr. Appel considers a major research recommendation to be investigating the effect of hydration status and fluid intake on chronic disease such as kidney stones and gallstones, as well as on the occurrence of specific cancers, including colon cancer and bladder cancer. From his perspective, a case can be made for conducting observational studies rather than trials to address this research recommendation.

Dr. Appel took the position that the recommendation to use large-scale surveys to validate estimates of total water intake (from food plus fluids) should be expanded to include the electrolytes and other nutrients. A comparison of potassium intakes that were reported in the Health Professionals Follow-up Study, the Nurses Health Study, and national survey data (IOM, 2005) reveals large differences. In view of this and of large absolute values reported at the upper quintiles of potassium intake, Dr. Appel suggests that the results of food frequency questionnaires be investigated for systematic bias.

Sulfate

No progress was reported related to the two research recommendations for sulfate, both of which call for studies of relationships between sulfate intake and specific disease conditions.

DRI Taxonomy and Process

The following comments relate to improving the DRI process.

Consideration of Chronic Disease

Dr. Appel concurred with Dr. Lupton that the process of applying the DRI model to chronic diseases needs further consideration. A related concern involves the definition of a healthy population, especially given the high probability of subsequently developing chronic disease. It could be that only 10 percent of people are healthy from the standpoint that they will never develop a problem with hypertension. In Dr. Appel's view, however, the public health problem is that 90 percent of people develop hypertension, and nutritional factors are related to its incidence.

Approaches to Setting Recommendations

Evidence-based medicine The most highly valued types of studies in evidence-based medicine—namely nutrition intervention trials with several doses and well-defined clinical outcomes—are rare for any nutrient. There are major impediments to conducting such studies.

Surrogate outcomes It often was necessary for DRI panels to use surrogate outcomes for setting nutrient recommendations. However, the criteria and process for selecting surrogate outcomes are ill defined and, in some cases, may have led to results that merit reconsideration.

Adequate Intake As illustrated for water, sodium, and potassium, different approaches were used to set the AI for each nutrient. It may be helpful to catalog the approaches used for setting the AI for different nutrients and consider revision to the definition.

Tolerable Upper Intake Level There is a need to consider ways to apply the DRI model for nutrients for which there is a direct progressive relationship between intake and the occurrence and/or severity of the adverse effect but for which there is no threshold. As illustrated by Figures 8-1 and 8-2, a threshold is not evident for either saturated fat or sodium intake.

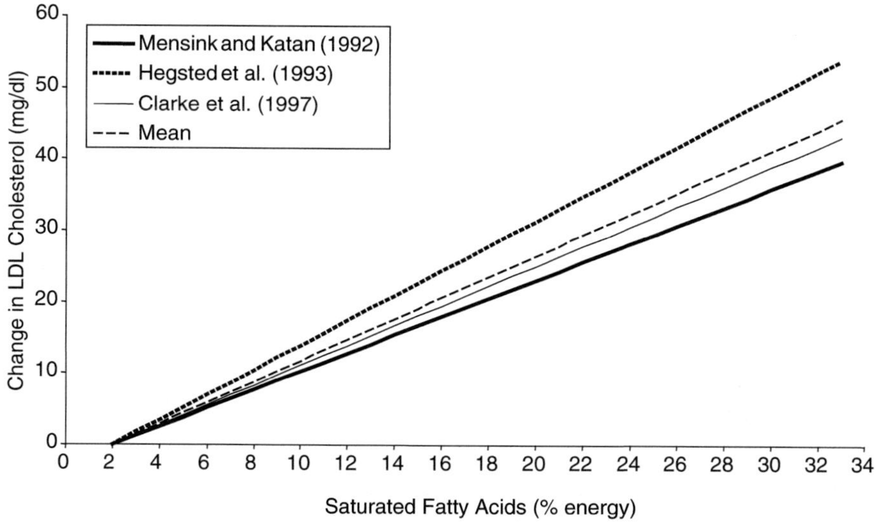

FIGURE 8-1 Calculated changes in serum low density lipoprotein cholesterol (LDL-C) concentration in response to percent change in dietary fatty acids.
SOURCE: IOM (2005).

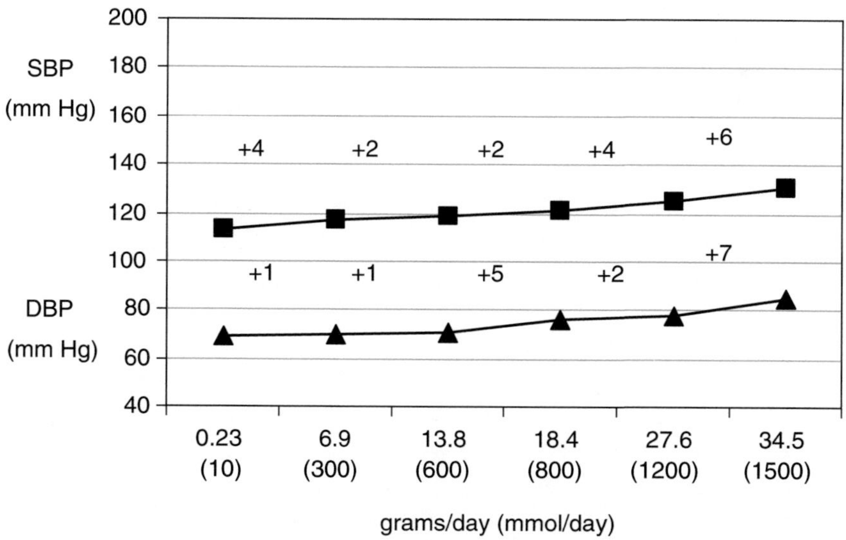

FIGURE 8-2 Increases in blood pressure observed in sodium dose–response trials.
NOTE: SBP = systolic blood pressure; DBP = diastolic blood pressure.
SOURCE: IOM (2005), with data from Luft et al. (1979).

Adjusting Nutrient Recommendations

Criteria are needed for determining whether adjustments need to be made in nutrient recommendations and for the kind of adjustment to make if one is needed. For example, should the specific type of DRI be based on calorie intake, weight, age, and/or sex? A major determinant of sodium intake is the number of calories consumed. A 4,000 kcal diet is likely to provide about twice as much sodium as a 2,000 kcal diet, but, as set, the AI does not take this into consideration.

Prioritizing Recommendations

A deliberate process is needed for writing and refining the research recommendations and then identifying the ones that are most likely to advance the field.

DISCUSSION

Tolerable Upper Intake Level for Potassium

In response to a request for a reason why a UL was not set for potassium, Dr. Appel clarified that no evidence of toxicity could be found for healthy people despite extensive searches, and that it would have been beyond the panel's charge to set a UL for the large number of people with chronic renal disease.

Ongoing Research

Dr. Dwyer asked whether the Chronic Renal Insufficiency Cohort (CRIC) Study might be a source of answers to some of the research questions raised. Dr. Appel noted that CRIC is an observational study, but that the need really is for some experimental evidence.

9

Dietary Reference Intakes for Infants and Children[1]

This session focused on major research needs related to the setting of Dietary Reference Intakes (DRIs) for infants and children. Lindsay H. Allen of the Western Human Nutrition Research Center at the University of California, Davis, who served on the Standing Committee on the Scientific Evaluation of Dietary Reference Intakes and is a former Food and Nutrition Board member, addressed major issues related to setting DRIs for infants and children. Nancy F. Krebs,[2] of the University of Colorado Health Sciences Center, a current Food and Nutrition Board member, focused on the use of zinc stable isotopes to inform the DRI process for these age groups.

SETTING DIETARY REFERENCE INTAKES FOR CHILDREN

Presenter: Lindsay H. Allen

This presentation covered three main topics: (1) a summary of the derivation of the DRIs for infants and children and of related problems that may be solvable, (2) issues that have been identified from the application of DRIs for children in various settings and their implications, and (3) the major knowledge gaps that were identified in the series of reports

[1]This chapter is based on a transcript and slides from the workshop.
[2]Dr. Krebs acknowledged contributions from K. Michael Hambidge, Leland V. Miller, Jamie Westcott, Lei Sian, and Xiaoyang Sheng.

and comments on whether those gaps can be filled. Information on the derivation of the DRIs was included to help clarify research gaps.

Derivation of DRIs for Infants

No Estimated Average Requirements (EARs) were set for infants because of lack of appropriate data. Adequate Intakes (AIs) were set instead. Thus, methods are lacking to estimate the prevalence of inadequate intakes or to plan complementary feeding for infants. This poses a large problem in developing countries where there may be a need for fortified foods.

Young Infants

The AI for all the nutrients for infants in the first six months of age was obtained by multiplying the average daily volume of breast milk (780 mL) times the concentration of the nutrient in breast milk. One serious problem is the accuracy of the data on human milk composition. The reported nutrient values for human milk vary widely among and within different studies. Reasons include small numbers of subjects, changes in composition over the course of feeding and over the course of lactation, improper sampling, effects of supplement use and food fortification on milk composition, and analytical problems. All these problems could be overcome.

A few examples illustrate the nature and extent of the limitations of data on human milk composition. For iron, the average concentration is said to be 0.35 mg/L, but the literature provides values ranging from 0.20 to 0.88 mg/L. The 0.35-mg value is approximately in the middle of that range. One new study from Sweden (Domellof et al., 2004), which has a large sample size relative to other studies, reports a value of 0.29 mg of iron per liter of breast milk, which, in practice, is considerably lower than the 0.35-mg value in current use. For vitamin A, an average of 485 μg/L is the value chosen, but the values considered ranged from 314 μg/L to 640 μg/L. The situation is similar for vitamin B_{12}, for which a value of 0.42 μg/L was chosen. The lowest reported value, 0.31 μg/L, was from vegans; the highest value, 0.91 μg/L, was from Brazilian women who received prenatal supplements. Folate analysis also has been very controversial. Dr. Allen emphasized that erroneous estimates of breast milk composition have a huge influence on the AIs during the first year after birth, and that this is a straightforward problem that could be remedied.

Older Infants

Several methods were used to derive the AI for infants in the second six months of age. When appropriate data were available, the AI was obtained by adding the estimated mean intake of the nutrient from solid food to the amount of that nutrient provided by 600 mL of breast milk. Dietary data on nutrients from solid foods were unavailable for many of the nutrients. Thus, in many cases, the AI was obtained by extrapolating up from the younger infants and/or down from older age groups (see "Extrapolation and Interpolation" section). The factorial method was used to set the AI for three nutrients, and a few other approaches were used as well. For example, serum 25-hydroxyvitamin D, or 25-(OH)D, concentration was used to set the AI for vitamin D, and that AI has since been questioned. In many cases, the values obtained using two or more methods were compared to examine face validity.

Derivation of DRIs for Children

Overview of Methods Used

Many different methods were used to set EARs, Recommended Dietary Allowances (RDAs), and AIs for children as follows:

- Energy (from birth; total energy expenditure plus growth)
- Protein (nitrogen balance, protein deposition)
- Linoleic, linolenic acids (breast milk plus median intake from the Continuing Survey of Food Intake by Individuals [CSFII])
- Vitamin D (from birth; serum 25-(OH)D)
- Calcium (factorial, balance)
- Phosphorus (factorial)
- Iron (factorial, assumes 10% bioavailability)
- Zinc (factorial)
- Fluoride (caries prevention)

- All others (extrapolation and/or interpolation)

If the value being extrapolated was an AI, the child value also must be an AI, with all its limitations. Some of these methods may not have produced reasonable values (for example, see presentation on zinc by Dr. Nancy Krebs).

Extrapolation and Interpolation

Questions have been raised about the approaches used for extrapolating DRI values from one age group to another. Examination of this issue calls for a description of the methods used.

- Extrapolation up from the AI for infants ages 0 to 6 months to obtain an AI for infants ages 7 to 12 months was usually based on body weight, using body weight to the 0.75 power to correct for surface area changes, which are large during that period of life.
- Extrapolation down from the adult EAR to the child EAR used the equation:

$$EAR_{child} = EAR_{adult} \times F$$

Where F = the following factor:

$$(weight_{child}/weight_{adult})^{0.75}\ (1 + \text{growth factor})$$

In this case the references weights were obtained from the Third National Health and Nutrition Examination Survey (NHANES III). Growth factors were based on the approximate proportional increase in protein requirements for growth (FAO/WHO/UNU, 1985). The growth factor value was 0.3 for children younger than 3 years of age and 0.15 for older children. These growth factor values were used for all the extrapolations, but they may not be appropriate for all nutrients because there is unevenness in the timing of the deposition of some nutrients. Some, such as protein and calcium, are deposited in large amounts during growth. Others, such as B vitamins, are not.

Before this workshop, Dr. Stephanie Atkinson of McMaster University in Ontario, Canada, provided Dr. Allen with comments on interpolation and extrapolation and how this has been done in other countries from 13 reports and 1 review. Her comments were based on the paper

Determining Life Stage Groups and Extrapolating Nutrient Intake Values prepared by Drs. Anderson and Koletzko for an international meeting on dietary recommended intakes. The report from that meeting will be available in 2007 in the United Nations University's *Food and Nutrition Bulletin.* Table 9-1 summarizes the approaches to extrapolation. Four major conclusions from the review are listed below:

1. Use the new World Health Organization growth standards for weight, length-for-height, and body mass index (BMI) for ages 0 to 5 years. (The Institute of Medicine [IOM] used height and BMI data from NHANES III and later from the Centers for Disease Control and Prevention [CDC] for interpolation and extrapolation.)
2. Base the extrapolation on body weight for nutrients that are not associated with metabolic rate.
3. Use body weight$^{0.75}$ for nutrients related to metabolic rate.
4. Base cutoff points for age categories on biology.

Derivation of Tolerable Upper Intake Levels

Vitamins A, D, and K, fluoride, selenium, zinc, and iron were the only nutrients for which reliable data were available on which to derive the Tolerable Upper Intake Levels (ULs). Most of the ULs for children were obtained by extrapolating the adult UL value down, based on body

TABLE 9-1 Extrapolations: Different Approaches

	Actual Weight	Reference Weight	Metabolic Weight	Energy	Interpolated
Canada/United States	X		X	X	
Caribbean	X				
Germany/Austria/ Switzerland	?				
European Union	X			X	X
Finland		X			
France	None?	⟶	⟶	⟶	⟶
Mexico	X				
United Kingdom	X?				

SOURCE: Atkinson and Koletzko, Determining Life Stage Groups and Extrapolating Nutrient Intake Values. Food and Nutrition Bulletin (in press).

weight. Dr. Allen stated that the ULs for children probably are relevant only to nutrients obtained from supplements. For infants and children, the UL is very close to the AI—particularly for vitamin A and zinc.

Problems Identified Upon Applying Selected Dietary Reference Intakes

Inconsistencies

Table 9-2 identifies nutrients for which the recommended intakes for 7- to 12-month-old infants are higher than those for 1- to 4-year-old children. These AIs were set by adding intake of the nutrient from complementary foods to the amount of the nutrient provided by 600 mL of breast milk. The reason for the inconsistency relates to the high content of specific nutrients in the complementary foods that were eaten by the 7- to 12-month-old U.S. infants. This inconsistency poses problems when trying to develop complementary food recommendations for developing countries.

Another inconsistency is a very large increase in recommended intake of some nutrients going from 7 to 12 months up to 1 to 3 years (Table 9-3). The basis for these large increases is unclear. In practice, the application of these recommended intake values is very difficult. Usually, the period of 6 months to 4 years is viewed as a continuum in infant feeding, not a time of sharp changes in nutrient needs.

TABLE 9-2 Inconsistency: Recommended Intakes for 7- to 12-Month-Old Infants Are Higher Than Those for 1- Through 3-Year-Old Children

	Recommended Intake, by Age Group	
Nutrient	7–12 months	1–3 years
Vitamin A (µg RAE)	500	300
Vitamin C (mg)	50	15
Iodine (µg)	130	90
Iron (mg)	11	7

NOTE: RAE = retinol activity equivalent.

TABLE 9-3 Inconsistency: Large Increases in Recommended Intakes Occur at Age 12 Months

	Recommended Intake, by Age Group	
Nutrient	7–12 months	1–3 years
Folate (μg)	80	150
Calcium (mg)	270	500
Phosphorus (mg)	275	460
Vitamin K (μg)	2.5	30

High Recommended Fiber Intakes

Following up on earlier comments about the AIs for fiber, Dr. Allen concurred that they probably are too high for children. Table 9-4 shows how the intake range for dietary fiber compares with the AI, by age group. Notably, the upper end of each range of reported intake is far below the AI. Dr. Allen asked, "Is it even possible to achieve the [fiber] AI in U.S. [and Canadian] children?"

Questionable Estimates of the Prevalence of Inadequacy

Despite the application of correct methods of analysis, some nutrients may be incorrectly identified as inadequate in the diets of children. Dr. Allen pointed out that there appears to be an inconsistency: 58 percent of the children ages 1 to 2 years in the CSFII had intakes less than the EAR for vitamin E, but fewer than 1 percent of them had inadequate intakes of any other nutrient (Devaney et al., 2004).

Similarly, nearly 80 percent of school children in the CSFII had intakes of vitamin E less than the EAR, 36 percent had intakes of magnesium less than the EAR, and 20 percent had intakes of phosphorus less than the EAR (Suitor and Gleason, 2002).

Although it has been suggested that the finding of a high prevalence of inadequacy of vitamin E might be a result of underestimation of vitamin E intakes (see Chapter 5 covering the DRIs for antioxidant nutrients), more information is needed on this topic. Do the findings for the U.S. school children suggest that the EARs for vitamin E, magnesium, and phosphorus are too high? Are inadequate intakes of vitamin E, phosphorus, and magnesium really the most common inadequacies in U.S. school children based on biological data?

TABLE 9-4 A Comparison of Dietary Fiber Intake with the Respective AI, by Age Group

Age (years)	AI (g/d)	Intake range (g/d)
1–3	19	5–12 [a]
4–8	25	6–18
9–13	26–31 [c]	9–11 [b]

[a]For 1- to 2-year-old children.
[b]For 10- to 12-year-old children.
[c]Value depends on individual's energy intake.

Very High Prevalences of Intakes Greater Than the UL

Analysis of CSFII intake data for certain nutrients has revealed a very high prevalence of intakes greater than the UL. For example, 90 percent of formula-fed infants ages 0 through 11 months exceed the UL for zinc, and 39 percent exceed the UL for vitamin A. High percentages of children ages 1 to 4 years exceeded the UL for zinc, vitamin A, and sodium, but less than 1 percent exceeded the UL for other nutrients. Do these findings represent a problem with intakes, the ULs, or both?

Knowledge Gaps Identified

In the full set of DRI reports, 43 knowledge gaps were identified that pertained to infants, children, and/or adolescents. Of these, 11 essentially said that studies are needed to set child and adolescent EARs for a range of vitamins using graded levels of intake and clearly defined cutoff points (i.e., biomarkers) for adequacy and inadequacy and that these studies should be conducted over a sufficient duration. With few exceptions, such studies have not been done at all. Thus, the question is, Is it feasible to address this research need relating to children?

Possible Approaches to Fill Knowledge Gaps

Vitamin Requirements

Some suggested approaches for improving knowledge of vitamin requirements include the following:

- Test responses to interventions in populations with a high prevalence of deficiency. Many studies have been conducted, and more are underway.
- Possibly feed the nutrient in doses slightly below and above the EAR long enough to see changes in biomarkers. This approach would be expensive, time-consuming, and difficult.
- Conduct studies with stable isotopes (e.g., deuterated retinol, deuterated vitamin D) or nanotracers (^{14}C-folate and ^{14}C-tocopherol, ^{14}C-vitamin B_{12}) by accelerator mass spectrometry.
- Stable isotope studies could be used for several purposes, including the following:
  - To estimate the percent absorption from breast milk and food
  - To conduct kinetic modeling (this requires a time series; for example, Haskell et al. [2004] used a population-based plasma kinetics approach to look at vitamin A stores and requirements in Peruvian children)
  - To estimate the intake that maintains pool size (see, for example, information on the paired deuterated-retinol-dilution technique [Haskell, et al., 2004])

Mineral Requirements

Studies with stable isotope tracers could improve knowledge of mineral requirements, for example:

- Measure bioavailability.
  - Absorption of ^{58}Fe from breast milk equals 16 percent in Swedish infants (Domellof et al., 2002).
  - Measure the effects of foods on breast milk iron absorption (Abrams et al., 2005) based on erythrocyte incorporation.
- Measure absorption, excretion, pool size, and turnover to determine requirements, as with zinc (Krebs et al., 2006).

Feasible ways to determine the intakes of calcium, phosphorus, magnesium, and vitamin D needed to maximize bone mineral accretion among 1- to 18-year-old children include the following:

- Studies of calcium, phosphorus, and magnesium balance and retention at varying levels of intake. Based on the adult experience, however, this work is expected to lead to questions about whether maximal retention is the appropriate approach to use with calcium, for example.

- Studies using stable isotopes of calcium and magnesium to measure absorption, pools, excretion, and so on. Abrams and colleagues (2005) reported on dual calcium isotope tracer and timed urine collection—a very rapid way to look at calcium absorption.
- More data are needed on relationships of vitamin D intake and serum 25-(OH)D with parathyroid hormone, bone turnover markers, immune function, and bone mineral density.

Although Dr. Allen indicated that the relationship between absorbed phosphorus and serum phosphorus probably could be determined, she questioned whether it is an important knowledge gap.

Macronutrients

Dr. Allen considers it feasible, timely, and important to address major knowledge gaps identified in the DRI Macronutrients Report (IOM 2002/2005) regarding activity factors for the management of body weight in children, total energy expenditure in children, measurement of the Physical Activity Level (PAL) in children, and diet composition patterns related to weight loss and accretion of lean tissue.

Electrolytes and Water

With regard to research recommendations in the DRI Electrolytes and Water Report (IOM, 2005), Dr. Allen considers it difficult to establish linkages of electrolyte needs and relationships of sodium and potassium in infancy with blood pressure and bone health later in life. Water turnover could be measured from the disappearance of deuterium from labeled water over time.

A Summary of Research Needs Related to Dietary Reference Intakes for Infants and Children

In conclusion, Dr. Allen identified the following research that needs to be conducted related to DRIs for children:

- More analysis of breast milk, collected appropriately
- If extrapolating, use new World Heath Organization standards
- More nutrient intake data (especially from complementary foods) related to biomarkers that are validated in children
- Studies with stable isotopes and nanotracers to determine vitamin and mineral bioavailability, kinetic studies, and possibly change in pool size on different vitamin intakes
- Doubly labeled water studies to measure energy expenditure and water turnover
- Determination of vitamin D requirements based on relationships of intake with 25-(OH)D, parathyroid hormone, bone markers, and so on

Although measuring food intake by infants and children is difficult, children need their own evidence-based DRIs. If DRI values for children are incorrect, this can result in incorrect identification of nutrient intake problems (either too little or too much), incorrect dietary recommendations for child feeding programs, and, potentially, adverse effects on health.

THE USE OF ZINC STABLE ISOTOPES TO INFORM THE DIETARY REFERENCE INTAKE PROCESS FOR INFANTS AND CHILDREN

Presenter: Nancy F. Krebs

This presentation focused on two major topics: (1) the use of zinc stable isotopes in the estimation of zinc requirements in infancy and (2) the DRI process for setting the zinc UL for infants and children. The related DRI research recommendation involves the need for quantitative data on human zinc homeostasis under a wide range of dietary conditions and at all ages (number 211-D).[3] The type of study identified as particularly useful for this purpose was the use of stable isotope methodology to quantify responses to changes in intake and absorption over a long term. The presentation included a review of stable isotope methodologies for zinc (including dosing, collections, and data); issues particular to infants and young children (invasiveness, collections, constraints on study design); and considerations for refining estimates of zinc requirements and revisiting the UL for zinc.

Advances in Understanding the Zinc Requirement

Studies of Zinc Homeostasis in Children

Figure 9-1 illustrates zinc homeostasis. Unlike other nutrients, a substantial amount of zinc is secreted into the gastrointestinal (GI) tract. Some of that zinc is reabsorbed, and some passes out into the stool. Urinary zinc content does not reflect dietary zinc intake. For infants and children, one needs to consider the accretion of zinc in new tissue.

The DRI micronutrients panel used the factorial approach to determine the physiologic requirement for zinc and thus as a basis for the EAR. The amount that is absorbed needs to cover the losses from all sources plus the amount needed to account for the accretion of zinc in new tissue. Therefore, it is necessary to obtain data on the amount of zinc absorbed over an entire day rather than from a single "test meal." Over the past few years, there has been a fundamental shift in the methods used to determine the physiologic requirement for zinc.

[3]See Appendix C for the exact wording of the recommendation that corresponds to the identification number given, and see Appendix D for the name of the report that corresponds to the letter.

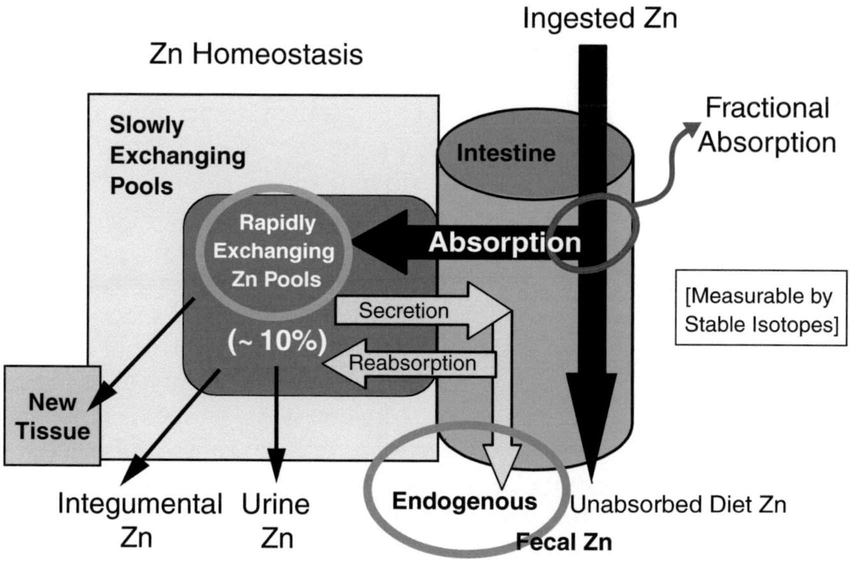

FIGURE 9-1 Diagram depicting zinc homeostasis.
NOTE: Zn = zinc.

Stable isotopes are useful for measurements mainly in the GI tract processes. Such measurements include the following:

- Fractional absorption—the proportion of ingested zinc that actually is getting into the system
- The excretion of endogenous zinc secreted into the GI tract
- Estimated size of the rapidly exchanging pool, which makes up about 10 percent of total body zinc

Despite considerable progress, much work still is needed in terms of validating what the findings really represent in terms of zinc status.

Stable Isotope Methodological Considerations

Historically, studies have posed many difficulties, two of which are collecting sufficiently large urine samples and complete fecal samples from infants, and avoiding contamination. Some advances that have been particularly relevant to being able to do studies with stable isotopes in children relate to using urine for measures of fractional absorption with the so-called dual isotope tracer ratio technique. The use of this technique provides multiple measurements to average, rather than just one end point. Better instrumentation allows the use of spot urine, greatly reducing collection demands. Three different stable isotopes of zinc are available and can be used concurrently to track different processes and to look at different conditions in the same person.

Fecal monitoring with an isotope of zinc plus the rare earth element dysprosium now makes it possible to measure the completeness of the fecal collection and also to obtain fractional absorption from a fecal sample more easily, without a requirement for an intravenous dose. Moreover, by using dysprosium in combination with isotopes and obtaining partial fecal and spot urine collections for 4 to 5 days, the endogenous fecal zinc excretion can be estimated.

Better instrumentation now allows the use of lower doses. The cost of isotopes has decreased dramatically in the past 10 years. Thus, the major cost is the labor involved in the analyses.

Examples of Applications of New Methods

In well-nourished individuals at the lowest doses of zinc, fractional absorption is very high; it decreases steadily with increases in the dose. The high fractional absorption of a low dose is not due to zinc deficiency. Instead, it is due to a very small amount of zinc in the GI tract. With a low dose, even though there is a high fractional absorption, the amount actually getting absorbed is small. There is essentially a linear relationship of dietary zinc to absorbed zinc at the lower doses. For aqueous doses of zinc in the postabsorptive state, at an intake of about 20 mg of zinc, the amount absorbed levels off.

Dr. Krebs' group has extended this work, done some pharmacokinetics modeling, used a saturation response model extensively, and applied findings to other data. Figure 9-2 is a plot of zinc intake versus absorbed zinc in young infants. Fractional absorption is high for breast-fed infants, but the amount absorbed remains less than that of formula-fed infants. The UL for this age group is 5 mg/day—less than the amount consumed by all but one of the formula-fed infants. This kind of plotting can be informative in terms of bioavailability and requirements.

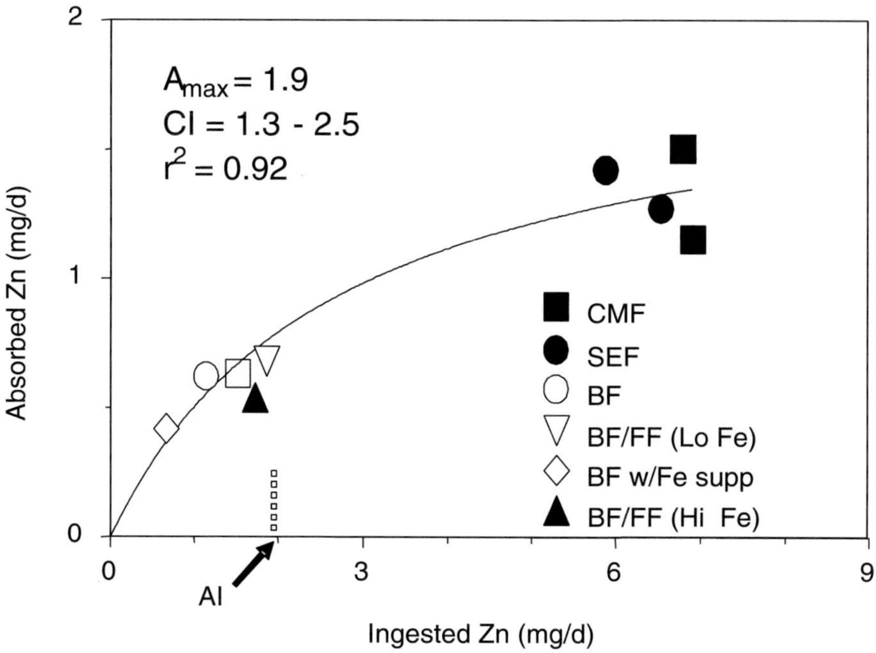

FIGURE 9-2 Zinc intake versus absorbed zinc in infants ages 2–4 months: Saturation response model.
NOTE: A_{max} = maximum absorption; CI = confidence interval; Zn = zinc; CMF = cow milk formula; SEF = semielemental formula; BF = breast-fed (exclusively); BF/FF = breast-fed with formula intake (6 oz/day); Lo Fe = 4 mg/L iron-fortified formula; Hi Fe = 12 mg/L iron-fortified formula; BF w/Fe supp = exclusively breast-fed with daily iron supplement (15 mg/day).
SOURCE: Adapted from Hambidge, et al (in press)

A plot of the endogenous fecal zinc versus absorbed zinc over a day shows a good correlation between the two. In Figure 9-3, the breast-fed infants are represented by the symbols on the left. Homeostatic mechanisms, including the conservation of endogenous zinc, enable the breast-fed infants to achieve positive net zinc absorption.

Absorption studies and application of the saturation–response curve to data provide information useful for predicting the effects of feeding different complementary foods to older infants, as shown in Figure 9-4. At 7 months of age, the breast milk alone provides less zinc than required. Feeding unfortified cereal is predicted to have little impact on the total amount of zinc absorbed. By adding meat (in this case, beef) one dramatically increases both zinc intake and absorbed zinc, thus meeting the physiologic requirement.

In the Zinc-Fortified Wheat Study in Peruvian Preschool Children (Lopez de Romana et al., 2005), absorption studies helped explain the lack of a statistically significant effect of treatment times duration. Zinc absorption studies of Chinese toddlers revealed that (1) homeostatic mechanisms were not enough to compensate for their low zinc intakes, (2) there is reason to suspect zinc deficiency, and (3) there is a need for intervention trials. Dr. Krebs indicated that examining intakes relative to the EAR may be quite useful in predicting absorption and, therefore, response to proposed interventions.

The effects of phytate intake on zinc absorption are complex. Dr. Krebs and coworkers are using a trivariate model to examine zinc absorption as a function of intakes of both dietary zinc and phytate (model not yet published).

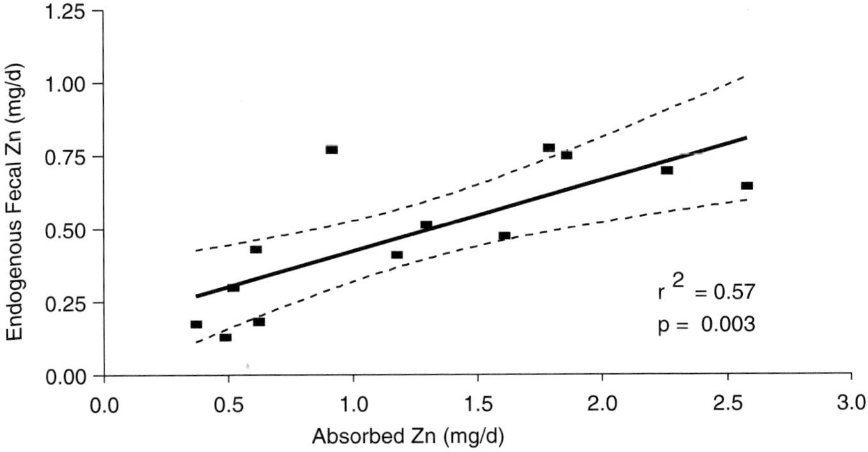

FIGURE 9-3 Absorbed zinc versus endogenous fecal zinc: breast-fed and formula-fed infants.
NOTE: Zn = zinc.
SOURCE: Krebs NF, Westcott JE. 2002. Zinc and breast-fed infants: If and when is there a risk of deficiency? In: Davis MK, Isaacs CE, Hanson LA, Wright AL, eds. Integrating Population Outcomes, Biological Mechanisms and Research Methods in the Study of Human Milk and Lactation. New York: Kluwar Academic/Plenum Publishers. With kind permission of Springer Science and Business Media.

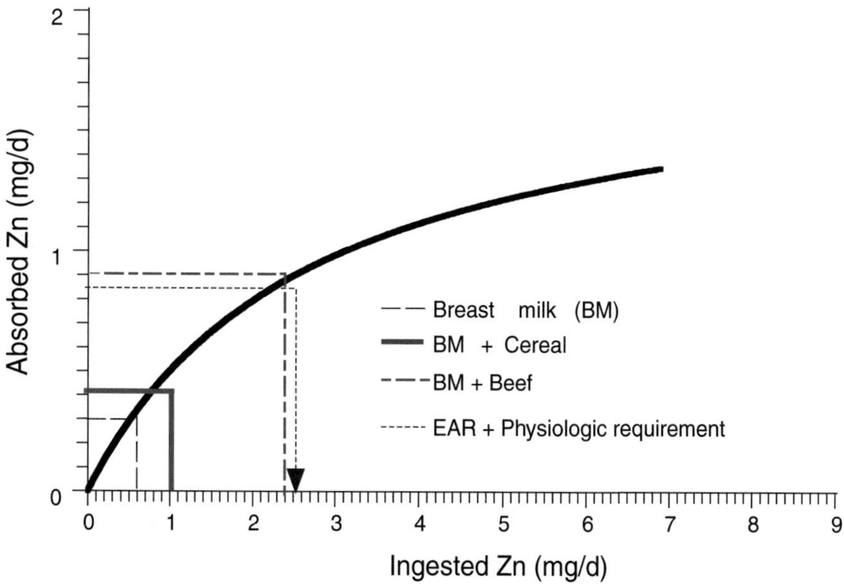

FIGURE 9-4 Absorbed zinc versus zinc intake at age 7 months: implications for complementary foods for breast-fed infants.
NOTE: EAR = Estimated Average Requirement.
SOURCE: Data from Hambidge et al., 2002; Jalla et al., 2006, Krebs et al., 2006

The DRI Process and the UL

More attention should have been given to intake assessment prior to setting the UL for zinc for young children, according to Dr. Krebs and Dr. Michael Hambidge, who served on the panel on micronutrients. As has been reported by many, a large proportion of infants and young children have zinc intakes that exceed the UL for zinc—largely because of infant formula and food fortification. Dr. Krebs took the position that there is no evidence that adverse effects have resulted, and she called for prompt amendment of the zinc UL to address this discrepancy.

Concluding Remarks

In conclusion, advances in stable isotope methodology have made it possible to conduct studies in diverse pediatric populations and settings. These methods can be taken to the field now. The application of stable isotopes to zinc homeostasis in infants and children suggest that

- absorption is characterized by a saturation–response model,
- the most important factors influencing zinc absorption are the quantity of zinc ingested and likely phytate (but not host status),
- homeostatic responses are insufficient to prevent dietary deficiency, and
- comparison of population intake to the current EAR for zinc seems to predict a response to interventions.

Furthermore, it is important to link homeostatic responses to interventions with functional outcomes.

DISCUSSION

Throughout the workshop, many discussions included mention of the serious data gaps related to setting EARs for infants and children. During this discussion, Dr. Bier called for the convening of experts to develop modeling approaches and other approaches to radiotracers in a way that advances the pediatric field. For example, there is the need for reduced sampling algorithms that allow compartmental modeling. How does one develop those reduced sampling algorithms? How can multiple tracers be used to develop time series?

Dr. Allen added that there is a big need to convene a group to examine methods that are most feasible, most ethical, and most convenient. Ethical considerations would include addressing the types of studies that should be allowable by institutional review boards.

10

Tolerable Upper Intake Levels[1]

This session presented perspectives on Tolerable Upper Intake Levels (ULs). Sanford A. Miller of the University of Maryland[2] provided the perspective of an individual who has observed the development of the Dietary Reference Intakes (DRI) program from its inception. He served as a member of the Upper Reference Levels Subcommittee, the Standing Committee on the Scientific Evaluation of Dietary Reference Intakes, and the Food and Nutrition Board. Christine Taylor of the Food and Drug Administration (FDA) recently completed a 2-year assignment to the World Health Organization (WHO); she provided perspectives based on a joint effort between the Food and Agricultural Organization (FAO) and WHO to describe a model for nutrient risk assessment.

TOLERABLE UPPER INTAKE LEVELS

Sanford A. Miller

This workshop reflects a concept underlying the development of the then new DRIs—that they would be in constant flux. Although some progress has been made over the last 10 years, an enormous amount remains to be done, especially with regard to providing the data needed to set the ULs. A search of the literature published over the last 6 years

[1]This chapter is based on a transcript and slides from the workshop.

[2]Patricia Anderson and Richard Forshee of the Center for Food, Nutrition, and Agriculture Policy at the University of Maryland provided input regarding progress made in filling the identified research gaps.

identified only about 30 papers that, even by a stretch of the imagination, could be used in revising or adding to the ULs. This presentation covers distinctions between risk and safety, several considerations for establishing ULs, data needs, and research needs.

Distinguishing Between Risk and Safety

To improve the process for setting ULs, it would be helpful to distinguish between risk and safety. *Risk* is an inherent property of a material. It depends upon exposure and a variety of factors, but it can be determined using scientific methods.

Safety, on the other hand, might be called a second order derivative of risk. Cultural, social, and other health reasons are used to decide what constitutes a safe dose. Safety must be defined, but it can be based on many factors other than scientifically based ones. Figure 10-1 illustrates this point.

In the DRI reports, the definition for UL is, "the highest level of daily nutrient intake that is likely to pose no risk of adverse health effects for almost all individuals in the general population." Dr. Miller asserted that for some nutrients this is a virtual impossibility. To eliminate the risk, one must set a very, very low value for the UL. In fact, one needs to set the UL so low that the intake would not provide the positive nutritional benefits of the nutrient. The UL for vitamin D provides an example of this. Thus, Dr. Miller's position is that the focus should be on *acceptable risk*, not *no risk.* Notably, ULs restrict dietary recommendations and regulatory policy options.

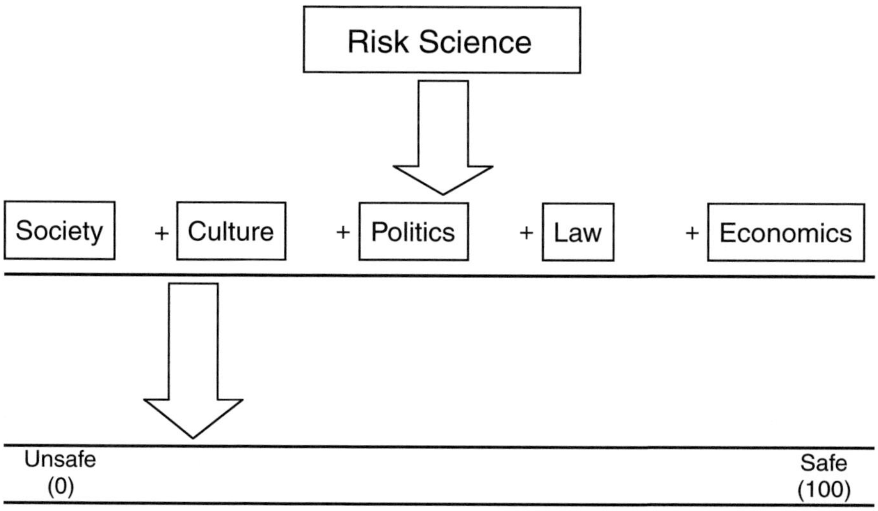

FIGURE 10-1 Safety: A point on a continuum.

Considerations in Establishing Tolerable Upper Intake Levels

Requirements to establish ULs include clear objectives, good models, and sufficient data. A clear objective would identify exactly what it is that is being protected against. Good models are needed to determine that protection is needed against a specified end point. Such models need to make it possible to calculate what exposures are going to be safe or not. However, the greatest need is for data.

Risk/Risk Model

To a large extent, the model that might be most useful is a risk/risk model. That is, what is the risk of having a very low UL versus a high UL? How does that interfere with other aspects of health? Instead, the DRI process has used the safe level model, while calling it a risk assessment model. Dr. Miller believes that the most useful approach will be some combination of risk/risk with a better understanding of biological mechanisms for the end points of concern.

Addressing Multiple End Points

An interesting aspect of nutrients is that multiple end points can be considered in a risk assessment—for example, end points concerned with a deficiency or the essentiality of the nutrient or other beneficial or adverse effects on health. Many nutrients are associated with several risk curves that show different risks with different intakes. Figure 10-2, developed with Dr. Richard Forshee for a hypothetical nutrient, depicts this situation. A reasonable public health goal is to recommend the consumption of the nutrient at a level that minimizes the total expected loss of health—the dotted line in Figure 10-2. Recommending a "safe level" (defined here as 0 expected loss of health) for either Risk 1 or Risk 2 would result in higher total expected loss of health than could be achieved by tolerating some risk from both Risk 1 and Risk 2. Modeling data in this way could help identify the intake at which the risks are minimized with regard to all aspects of the nutrient, and it may be the easiest way to minimize risk.

Data Needs

Data needs related to ULs are the same as they were 10 years ago:

- Dose–response information
- The ability to draw curves to determine the fundamental association between the substance and the outcome
- The potential toxicity or adverse effects of high intakes of nutrients on children
- Better measures of exposure
- The extent of the exposure in subpopulations
- The upper percentiles of consumption
- Long-term exposure data

Despite the many years that nutrition research has been conducted in animals and humans, there is virtually no information on what happens when humans exceed the requirement by 100-fold or 10-fold in order to prevent deficiency for a lifetime. The gold standard needs to be human exposure. Biomarkers are greatly needed to make it possible to conduct the kinds of human experiments that could provide better data for setting ULs.

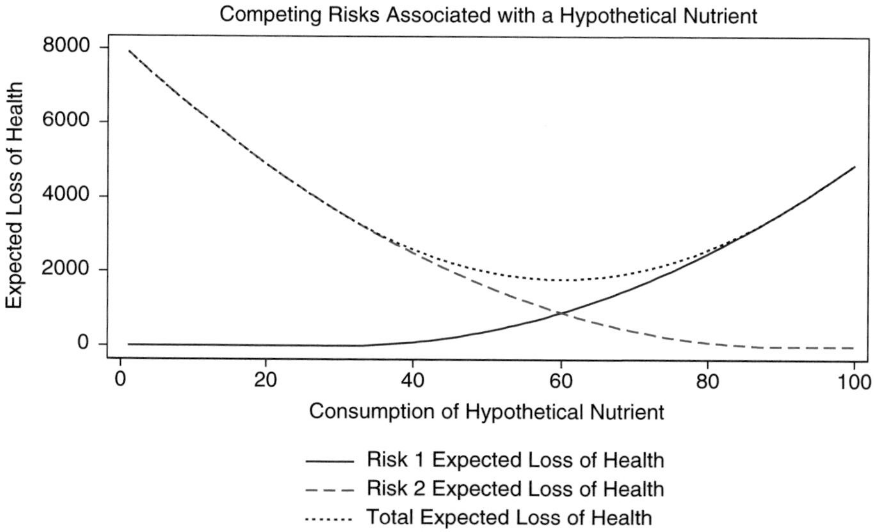

FIGURE 10-2 Two hypothetical risks and the total risk associated with consumption of a nutrient.
NOTE: This figure illustrates a hypothetical relationship in which consumption of a certain nutrient is associated with two risks that move in opposite directions as consumption of the nutrient increases. The vertical axis of this figure represents the expected loss of health in some standard unit, such as lives or quality-adjusted life years. The scale of the vertical axis is arbitrary and is intended for illustrative purposes only. The goal is to minimize the expected loss of health, that is to be as close to zero (0) on the vertical axis as possible. The horizontal axis represents the relative consumption of the nutrient from none (0) to the maximum observed consumption (100). The solid line represents expected loss of health from Risk 1. The expected loss of health from Risk 1 increases as consumption of the nutrient increases. The classic example of such a risk is toxicity at high levels of exposure, such as renal disease and vitamin D. The dashed line represents the expected loss of health from Risk 2. The expected loss of health from Risk 2 decreases as consumption of the nutrient increases. The classic example of this type of risk is a deficiency disease related to a nutrient, such as osteoporosis and vitamin D. The dotted line represents the total expected loss of health (sum of the expected losses from Risk 1 and Risk 2).

Research Needs

Among the many research needs identified by Dr. Miller are the following:

- *Translation of animal data to human health outcomes.* This requires knowledge of the mechanisms.
- *Chronic studies.* Although it is difficult to study chronic disease outcomes, more studies on such outcomes are needed to reduce important knowledge gaps.
- *Prioritization and communication of the research needs.*
- *Understanding of the interactions of multiple nutrients and health end points.* In terms of toxicity or adverse effect, examination of the interactions among various nutrients is an important part of the process of trying to determine safety.
- *Improved risk/risk models.* Data are needed on the risks of two different materials in a single food and differences in the risks of a single nutrient under various circumstances.

UPPER LEVEL RESEARCH RECOMMENDATIONS WITHIN THE CONTEXT OF AN INTERNATIONAL MODEL FOR NUTRIENT RISK ASSESSMENT

Presenter: Christine Taylor

This presentation addressed UL research recommendations from the perspective of work conducted recently by the WHO in cooperation with the FAO. The work resulted in the release of report of a Joint FAO/WHO Scientific Workshop on Nutrient Risk Assessment (FAO/WHO, 2005), which is available online at http://www.who.int/ipcs/methods/nra/en/index.html. The report fulfills a WHO and FAO role in providing scientific advice and is consistent with the WHO efforts to harmonize risk assessment methodologies. Five member states funded the workshop, which included 18 participants from 14 countries. The focus was on risk from excessive intake of nutrient substances; risk from deficiency was outside the scope of the workshop.

The workshop participants initially considered two types of information: (1) existing principles for risk assessment of nonnutrients and (2) the major published comprehensive quantitative nutrient risk assessment documents—mainly reports issued by three authoritative bodies from the European Union, the United Kingdom, and the United States and Canada (i.e., the Institute of Medicine [IOM]). The workshop participants then worked to develop a model for nutrient risk assessment, keeping in mind the distinction between nutrient risk assessment and nutrient risk management. Participants were not asked to develop specific upper levels[3] of intake for nutrient substances.

Considerations for a Model for Upper Levels

Principles that have evolved for conducting nonnutrient risk assessment offer the foundation for the model that appears in the WHO report. Those principles are modified, however, for special considerations related to nutrient substances, such as the following:

- One-of-a-kind homeostatic mechanisms
- Metabolic differences for age, sex, and life stage
- Dual risk curves—deficiency and excess
- Need to deal with inadequate data sets

The nutrient risk assessment model has at least three underlying themes:

1. Outcomes are based on available evidence, even if it is limited, not on "developed data sets."
2. The current practice of evidence-based systematic review needs to be adapted for relevance to nutrient risk assessment.
3. Public health protection decisions drive the process; choices are not necessarily based solely on considerations of the weight of the evidence.

Two general research messages evolved: (1) the need for research to improve the ability of risk assessors to deal with currently limited data sets, and (2) the need for research targeted very specifically to safety.

---

[3]The term *upper levels* is the term used in the FAO/WHO report. Its definition differs somewhat from the definition for the Tolerable Upper Intake Level (UL). Use of the abbreviation *UL* in the summary of Dr. Taylor's presentation is reserved for applications to the Dietary Reference Intakes.

Moreover, the workshop participants identified the need to develop ways to stimulate, organize, focus, and promote research agendas in this area.

Research Recommendations

The FAO/WHO report contains many research recommendations. Dr. Taylor organized these recommendations into seven themes for the purpose of this presentation:

1. Existing data sets
2. The need for human intervention data
3. Relevant measurable end points
4. Improving basic understanding
5. Improving and harmonizing dietary intake assessments
6. Adapting the model to a range of nutrient substances
7. Understanding uses of upper levels and of risk characterization

Overall, the research recommendations underscore comments made earlier in this DRI workshop that there is a need to consider the process for establishing upper levels of intake—not just for more data. Research messages organized under the seven themes follow, and, where applicable, their correspondence with recommendations from DRI reports is noted.

Dealing with Existing Data Sets

The workshop participants found the existing reports on nutrient risk assessment lacking in transparency regarding the scientific judgments made and reasons for the decisions made. The participants regarded the practice of scientific judgments to be a researchable area and thus the report calls for guidelines for approaches to scientific judgment (establishing upper levels is a researchable issue), and for specific efforts as part of nutrient risk assessment to incorporate accountability, documentation, and transparency.

Examples of improved methods for dealing with existing data sets include (1) defined approaches to combining data to establish links to adverse health effects, (2) inclusion/exclusion criteria for and weighting of studies (most of which are observational), and (3) enhanced principles for meta-analysis.

Dealing with the Need for Human Intervention Data

Although it was emphasized that limited human data sets should not remain the norm, the ability to fulfill research needs faces certain ethical issues as well as the costs and difficulties associated with human trials and intervention studies. Because of these challenges, there is a need to do the following:

- Develop innovative methodologies including animal models, in-vitro techniques, and computer simulations
- Explore more fully at least three areas:

  1. Approaches for comparing sensitivity between animals and humans
  2. Extrapolation of data from adults to children using approaches that are more physiological and less the default
  3. Relevance of changes in easily measured homeostatic mechanisms

DRI research recommendations related to this theme focused on adjustment factors for body size, physical activity, intakes of energy, and so on (433-G).[4]

Identifying Relevant Measurable End Points

Under this theme, emphasis was placed on causally related biomarkers:

- Identify, elucidate, and validate the biomarkers.
- Specify sensitivity.
- Clarify homeostatic range.
- Clarify time course.

---

[4]See Appendix C for the wording of the recommendations that correspond to the identification numbers given, and see Appendix D for the name of the report that corresponds to each letter.

One relevant DRI research recommendation was related to biomarkers (124-C).

Improving Basic Understanding

This is a very critical topic but challengingly broad. Work is needed to do the following:

- Elucidate the nature of metabolism, especially at high levels of intake.
- Target research to elucidate adverse health effects.
- Ensure the inclusion of dose–range studies and conduct more of them.
- Specify interactions.
- Establish bioavailability.

The topics above are similar to some of the research recommendations from the DRI reports, specifically:

- General research (420-G)
- Specific nutrients, including:
  - B vitamins, folate, pantothenic acid, and choline
  - Vitamin C, vitamin E, and carotenoids
  - Vitamin K, arsenic, boron, copper, molybdenum, silicon, and vanadium (supplements)
  - Amino acids and protein
- Dose–response data (421-G)
- Factors affecting uptake and absorption (456-H)

Improving and Harmonizing Dietary Intake Assessments

In the comparison of the three major risk assessments, a major source of inconsistencies was in the approach to dietary intake assessment. Thus, the FAO/WHO Working Group considered ways in which dietary intake assessment methods could be harmonized. Research needs include:

- Strategies for combining data to estimate intake from all sources

- Strategies for estimating intake from aggregated data—essential in many parts of the world that lack intake data on individuals
- Development of markers of exposure

DRI research recommendations related to this theme include quantification of the intake of dietary supplements (426-G), enhancement of food composition databases (435-G), and statistical adjustments (438-G).

Adapting the Model to a Range of Nutrient Substances

The substances that are to be included under the term *nutrients and related substances* were not specifically defined during the FAO/WHO workshop, but the term was intended to include a wide range of nondrug substances. This poses some difficulties in working with a risk assessment model. For example:

- Some nutrient substances are nonessential or nonbeneficial, but they are constituents of the food supply. Is the risk assessment model equally applicable to essential and nonessential nutrient substances?
- Some nutrient substances have no threshold response. These include trans fat and saturated fat. How does the model need to be adapted or modified for such nutrient substances?
- Is the model applicable to macronutrients and micronutrients?
- How can the model address interactions?
- How does one handle any apparent overlap that may be observed regarding "beneficial" intake and risk?

DRI research recommendations related to this theme covered the optimal range for macronutrient intake (255-E), nature of their adverse effects (261-E), and fats (343-E).

Understanding the Use and Application of the Upper Level and of Risk Characterization

This theme is on the border between risk assessment and risk management. The nature of the dialogue between risk assessors and risk managers is very important internationally. It may include iterative discussions because the risk assessor's actions must be very germane to the needs of the risk manager, but the risk assessor should avoid going beyond assessment into management decisions. The FAO/WHO Working Group called for studies of risk characterization outcomes to identify the following:

- What information was used and how? How could the information be improved?
- What aspects of characterization were not useful?
- What aspects led to secondary risk assessment requests?

The report also called for guidelines for problem formulation.

Concluding Points

With regard to public health protection, stakeholders provided comments emphasizing the importance of defining what is adverse. Clear terminology is of special importance when nutritionists and toxicologists are collaborating.

The process of selecting the critical adverse health effect for setting the upper level differed among the three authoritative bodies. The selection of a different critical adverse effect often produced different results in the setting of upper levels. According to the FAO/WHO nutrient risk assessment report, when there is an array of truly adverse health effects, one examines the end points from a public health protection filter and selects the effect seen at the lowest level of intake. The focus is not necessarily on the effect that is most severe or even the effect for which the weight of the evidence is strongest. This approach may lead to "conceptually messy" outcomes. Thus, much work needs to be done related to the selection of the critical adverse health effect and what it means in terms of coming up with appropriate and responsive upper levels.

Looking to the future, it may be advisable for the IOM to consider its role in international harmonization. One of the recommendations in the

FAO/WHO report is to create, expand, and/or combine databases to catalog and collate information.

DISCUSSION

In response to a query from Dr. Hathcock, Dr. Taylor clarified that the Highest Observed Intake Level was identified in the report as a way of assisting risk managers. The FAO/WHO Working Group was aware of the need to ensure that risk assessment outcomes were usable by risk managers. Participants recognized that failing to set an upper level in the face of insufficient data was problematic because risk managers often must make regulatory decisions that provide some measure of safety. Thus, the Highest Observed Intake Level was suggested as a way of providing some scientific context for such decisions.

Dr. Hathcock reiterated his previous concern that anomalous regulatory policies sometimes develop if an upper limit is not set. He hopes to help prevent illogical and inconsistent risk management decision making.

Dr. Miller commented that this is an important communications issue. People who are not particularly sophisticated or trained in risk assessment need to translate the assessment into policies or actions. Without an understanding of the differences, the lack or presence of a numerical value for the upper level can make the difference in the credibility of the particular policy or action. So this suggestion by the FAO/WHO Working Group to set a Highest Observed Intake Level is an important recognition of a communication problem.

In response to a question by Dr. Murphy regarding whether the high preformed vitamin A intake by infants is a problem, Dr. Krebs commented on the ULs for vitamin A and for zinc. In particular, Dr. Krebs indicated that she has no perception that the infants and children with the high reported intakes are experiencing any toxicity from those intakes, but that this question has not really been examined closely for either vitamin A or zinc. Dr. Krebs stated that she has no real basis for knowing. The saturation–response curves for zinc suggest that there is much more zinc in formula than is necessary, and the same may be true for iron.

In the final comment, Dr. Allen encouraged the use of metabolomics as a promising method to look at effects of toxic substances and of nutrition interventions. One can easily see large changes and a very large number of biomarkers upon changing the intake of a single nutrient.

11

Dietary Reference Intakes: Applications in Dietary Assessment and Planning[1]

In this session on the Dietary Reference Intakes (DRIs) application reports, five individuals addressed research recommendations related to dietary assessment and planning. Suzanne P. Murphy of the University of Hawaii (the first chair of the Subcommittee on Interpretation and Uses of Dietary Reference Intakes) covered research recommendations in the DRI Dietary Assessment Report (IOM, 2000a). Susan I. Barr of the University of British Columbia (the second subcommittee chair) covered research recommendations in the DRI Dietary Planning Report (IOM, 2003a). Jay Hirschman of the Food and Nutrition Service, Patricia M. Guenther of the Center for Nutrition Policy and Promotion, and Rena Mendelson of Ryerson University, Toronto, presented perspectives of users of the reports.

DIETARY REFERENCE INTAKES: APPLICATIONS IN DIETARY ASSESSMENT

Presenter: Suzanne P. Murphy

Dietary Reference Intakes: Applications in Dietary Assessment (IOM, 2000a) has been available for 6 years. This presentation summa-

[1]This chapter was written based on transcripts and slides from the workshop. Drs. Murphy and Barr each acknowledged input from several subcommittee members. Dr. Guenther acknowledged input by fellow members of the National Cancer Institute's Measurement Errors and Surveillance Working Group and the U.S. Department of Agriculture Center for Nutrition Policy and Promotion DRI Working Group.

rized the progress on the research recommendations. For convenience, the report's 29 research recommendations are grouped into four broad categories:

1. Improvements to the DRIs themselves
2. Improvements in dietary assessment methods
3. Better statistical methods
4. Tools to help professionals use the DRIs correctly

A brief discussion of each category follows, along with highlights of 12 of the general recommendations (the recommendations are italicized).

Recommendations That Were Related to the DRIs Themselves

Most of the recommendations have been covered by previous speakers, but they are summarized below along with Dr. Murphy's assessment of the progress made in reducing the research gap.

- *Obtain better data on the distribution of requirements.* To determine the Recommended Dietary Allowance (RDA), one needs some information on the variability of requirements. Many assumptions were necessary, and there is still a need to improve those estimates. Little progress has been made.
- *Replace Adequate Intakes (AIs) with Estimated Average Requirements (EARs) and RDAs.* Figure 11-1 depicts the possible placement of a "mythical" AI on a graph showing the frequency distribution of individual requirements. When the DRI nutrient panels did not have enough information to set an EAR and an RDA, they set this single number—the AI. Because one doesn't know anything about the distribution of requirements, one cannot use the paradigm that was developed for estimating the probability of adequacy or the prevalence of inadequacy. One only can look at whether mean intakes are at the AI. In most cases, the AI probably is larger than the RDA. Therefore, the AI is not a very satisfactory DRI value in terms of dietary assessment. Based on previous presentations during this workshop, some good progress is anticipated on replacing some of the AIs with EARs as time goes by.

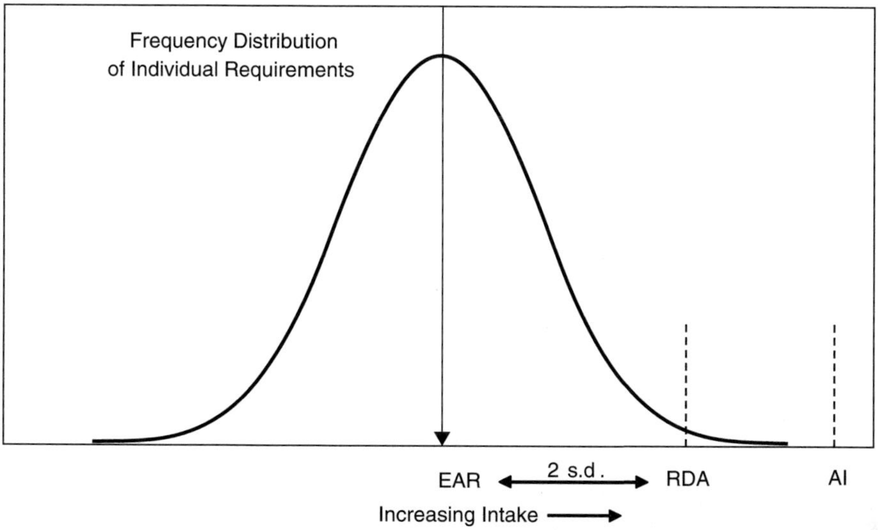

FIGURE 11-1 Position of selected DRI values on a frequency distribution of individual requirements.
NOTE: EAR = Estimated Average Requirement, RDA = Recommended Dietary Allowance, AI = Adequate Intake, s.d. = standard deviation. RDA = EAR + 2 s.d.

- *Set Tolerable Upper Intake Levels (ULs) for all nutrients and provide information on the distribution of adverse effects.* This type of distribution was not specified for any nutrient. If someone has an intake above the UL, one does not know if the risk of an adverse effect is very low or if there is great reason for concern. Little progress has been made.
- *Better specify factors that can alter requirements.* It could be useful to know if there were some way to determine approximately where on the requirement distribution a person's individual requirement falls. For example, Dr. Dawson-Hughes mentioned that the calcium requirement for children or for adolescents may be related to their height. Knowledge of such factors could be very helpful in estimating the probability of inadequacy for a specific person. Some progress is anticipated.

Recommendations Related to Improvement in Dietary Assessment Methods

Much work is being done in this area, as highlighted below.

- *Improve food composition tables to use the same units and forms as the DRIs.* This essentially has been accomplished, largely because of work by the Nutrient Composition Laboratory at the U.S. Department of Agriculture (USDA). For example, the food composition tables now list micrograms of dietary folate equivalents (μg of DFE). Alpha-tocopherol equivalents had to be changed to alpha-tocopherol, and in many databases the different tocopherols had not been separated out. Retinol equivalents had to be changed to retinol activity equivalents to adjust for the lower availability of some of the carotenoids. Also, the databases needed to include different forms of some nutrients for the EAR and the UL. For example, the UL for folate applies only to folic acid (the synthetic form of folate), whereas the EAR is for total folate and DFEs.
- *Improve dietary data collection instruments to remove the bias of underreporting.* This bias has long been recognized as one of the most serious problems with dietary assessment methods. Progress is being made. For example, the automated multiple pass method that is being used for U.S. national surveys seems to reduce underreporting and appears to be capturing much better data. Additionally, a group at the National Cancer Institute (NCI) is looking at a combination of recalls and a propensity questionnaire, a type of food frequency questionnaire to estimate the distribution of intakes for groups Additionally, the Observing Protein and Energy Nutrition (OPEN) Study that NCI conducted provided a much better understanding of the errors that are inherent in some dietary data.
- *Find better ways to quantify intakes from dietary supplements.* Considerable work is in progress on this topic. For example, 2 days of supplement intake data are being collected in U.S. national surveys, and this will provide some information on day-to-day variation in supplement intake. The USDA Nutrient Data Laboratory is building an analytic database so that it will become unnecessary to rely on label data. At the University of Hawaii, Dr. Murphy is conducting a study to try to quantify the errors in

reporting across multiple instruments used for collecting data on dietary supplements. It is hoped the findings will provide useful information about the accuracy of the data being collected.

Recommendations for Better Statistical Methods

Little progress has been made with regard to any of the research recommendations in this category, as described below.

- *Improve methods of assessing individuals.* Dr. Murphy noted that the use of the DRIs to assess an individual's intake is a highly contentious issue. Because a practical and valid process for determining an individual's usual intake is not yet available, reliance must be placed on estimates from reported intake or observed intake; and the resulting confidence in the assessment of adequacy may be low. Adjustment for the confidence of adequacy has been problematic; methods are not complete for all nutrients (that is, for nutrients with a high coefficient of variation of daily intakes), and the process is subject to misinterpretation (consumers and professionals may assume that a low confidence means that intake needs to be increased, but often it just means that intake needs to be observed over a longer period).

  Figure 11-2 presents a hypothetical example in which the EAR is 6.8, the RDA is 9, and the person's usual intake (based on the 3 days of intake data) is 10 units of this nutrient. If one simply calculates the straight probability of adequacy, the result would be about 100 percent; that is, if true usual intake were 10 units a day, one would be virtually certain that the individual met his or her requirement. However, the method used in the DRI Assessment Report also considers the uncertainty in basing the estimate of usual intake on only 3 days of reported intake. "True" usual intake could be either higher or lower than 10 units. In this situation, one would have much less confidence that the individual's true usual intake actually had 100 percent probability of adequacy. By using statistical equations and looking at the day-to-day variation in intake of the specific nutrient, the estimated confidence might be only 80 percent. Although the methods are quite good if one knows usual long-term diet, little progress has been made in improving the assessment methods for individuals for whom just a few days' data are available.

- *Assess the performance of the main methods of assessing groups, namely the full probability approach versus the cut-point method.* The cut-point method is much easier to apply than is the full probability approach, and it provides a very good approximation of the prevalence of inadequacy if the assumptions made are correct. The recommendation to conduct a systematic investigation of those assumptions has not yet been acted upon.

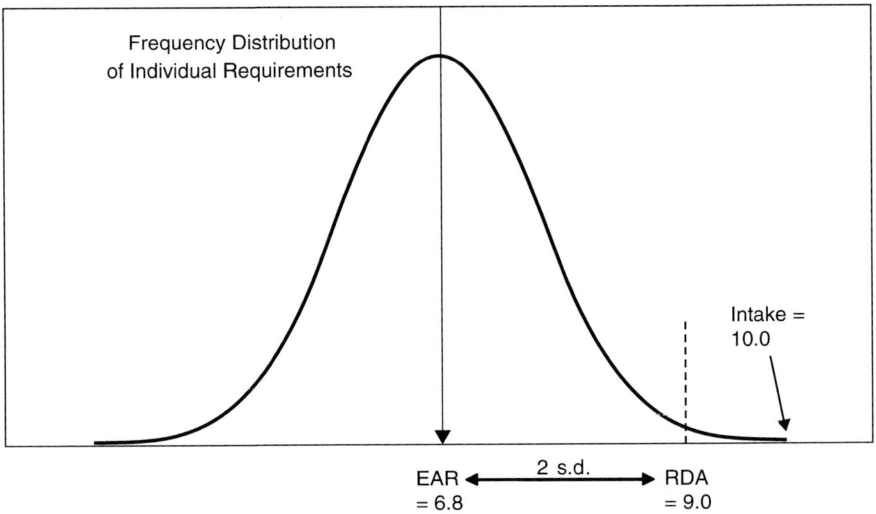

FIGURE 11-2 A usual long-term intake of 10.0 units would be above the RDA for this hypothetical nutrient and thus would have a high probability of adequacy. However, if intake data were available for only 3 days, then 10.0 might be higher or lower than the true usual intake, and the confidence that usual long-term intake was adequate would be reduced to approximately 80 percent.

NOTE: EAR = Estimated Average Requirement, RDA = Recommended Dietary Allowance, s.d. = standard deviation.

- *Develop methods to test for differences in the prevalence of adequacy between groups, controlling for other factors.* Suppose, for example, that one wanted to compare the prevalence of adequacy of nutrient intakes of two groups: (1) food stamp participants and (2) food stamp-eligible persons who were not participating in the program. To determine whether the results were statistically different, one would first have to adjust each distribution of intakes to obtain the usual intake distribution. Because the two groups may differ in other ways (e.g., income, education), multivariate analyses would be needed to adjust for the covariates. The DRI Assessment Report (IOM, 2000a) contains a proposed methodology to adjust for day-to-day variation and for these covariates, but it appears that the method has not been tested yet.[2]

Recommendations to Develop Tools to Help Professionals Use the DRIs Correctly

Some progress has been made with regard to extending software to assist users with new methods, but more and better tools are needed. The C-SIDE[3] program from Iowa State University is very helpful in assessing groups, but it is a rather complex program. A few of the software developers that have programs for assessing the diets of individuals have incorporated probability calculations into their programs rather than reporting intake as a percentage of the RDA.

---

[2]During discussion, Dr. Kevin Dodd, a statistician at NCI, clarified that the NCI statistical methodology can incorporate covariates. In looking at differences in nutrient intake among subpopulations, the NCI method holds potential for incorporating analytically the individual level covariates that can help predict usual intake. Those covariates could be from another instrument, from demographic data, and so on. A better prediction of individual intake will help in determining statistically significant differences in the distribution of usual intake within group, and the NCI group is working on that method.

[3]http://cssm.iastate.edu/software/side.html.

APPLICATIONS IN DIETARY PLANNING

Presenter: Susan I. Barr

The report *Dietary Reference Intakes: Applications in Dietary Planning* (IOM, 2003a) has been available for only 3 years. This presentation included an overview of the DRIs in planning and a summary of relevant research recommendations and progress to date.

Framework for Planning

The planning framework that was outlined in the DRI Planning Report provides some context for considering the research recommendations and the progress that has occurred. Figure 11-3 presents the conceptual framework for the uses of DRIs. It illustrates that to plan or assess diets, one needs valid estimates of nutrient requirements and of nutrient intakes. That is, planning and assessing are iterative processes: assessment is necessary for the planning, and planning needs be evaluated by assessment. The procedures used differ somewhat.

The goal stated for dietary planning is to optimize the prevalence of diets that are nutritionally adequate without being excessive. For an individual, the goal would be (1) a low risk that the person does not meet his or her individual requirement and (2) a low risk that the person's intake is excessive. For a group, this translates to a low prevalence of inadequacy and of potential risk of excess. Within this framework, planning goals are for intakes. Traditionally, however, planning has been for foods offered or served. In the DRI planning framework, what matters is not that the nutrient is available but whether or not it is consumed by the individual or group.

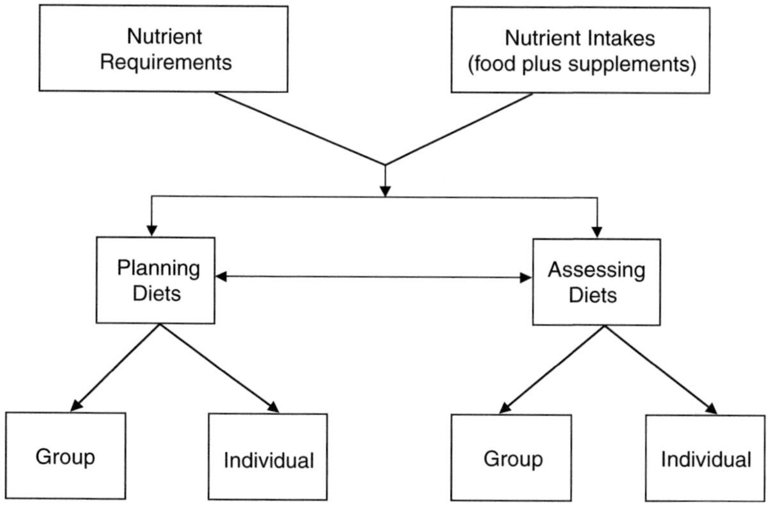

FIGURE 11-3 Conceptual framework: uses of Dietary Reference Intakes.
SOURCE: IOM (2000a), adapted from Beaton (1994).

An outline of the planning processes that the DRI Applications Subcommittee developed will help illuminate the research recommendations. Figure 11-4 illustrates the process used in planning for individuals. In this case, the relevant question is whether the individual has special considerations. If there were special considerations that would affect requirements (for example, smoking cigarettes increases the vitamin C needs of a smoker), then planning for that nutrient would be based on the special consideration. Planning for the other nutrients involves planning to meet the RDA or AI while keeping intake below the UL, meeting energy needs, and staying within the Acceptable Macronutrient Distribution Ranges (AMDRs).

Figure 11-5 shows the planning paradigm for groups. If the group is homogeneous (for example, a group of adult men), then one considers whether the requirement distribution is symmetrical or skewed. If it is not skewed, the plan can be based on the EAR cut-point method in such a way that the distribution of intake would have a low prevalence of persons with intakes below the EAR. If the requirement distribution were skewed, the full probability method would be used to achieve a low prevalence of inadequacy.

In the case of a heterogeneous group, the term *vulnerable subgroup* refers to a group that has a high nutrient requirement relative to energy needs. An example would be 6- to 12-month-old infants: they have high iron needs relative to their energy needs and could be a target for intervention.

A nutrient density approach to planning was proposed for heterogeneous groups for which vulnerable subgroups cannot be identified. This approach considers the joint distributions of energy and nutrient requirements to plan for the nutrient density that will lead to a low prevalence of inadequacy.

Figure 11-6 depicts the difference between the baseline usual intake distribution (dashed line) and the target usual intake distribution (solid line). The planning approach was used to attempt to shift the distribution to the right to lower the prevalence of inadequacy. Thus, in this target distribution, the prevalence of inadequacy (area to the left of the EAR) is now low, and usual intakes remain below the UL.

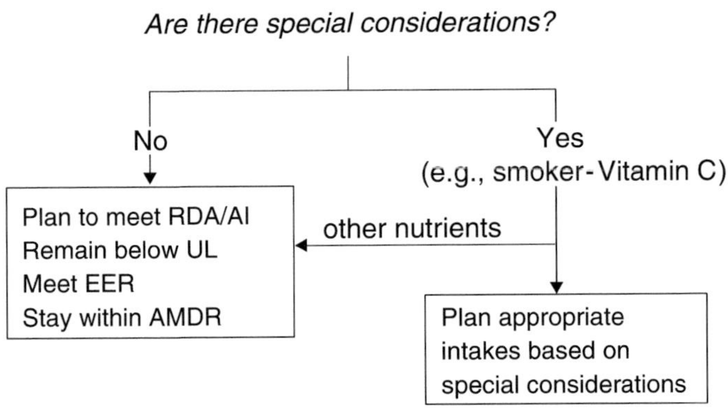

FIGURE 11-4 Decision tree for use when planning intakes for individuals. NOTE: RDA = Recommended Dietary Allowance, AI = Adequate Intake, EER = Estimated Energy Requirement, AMDR = Acceptable Macronutrient Distribution Range.

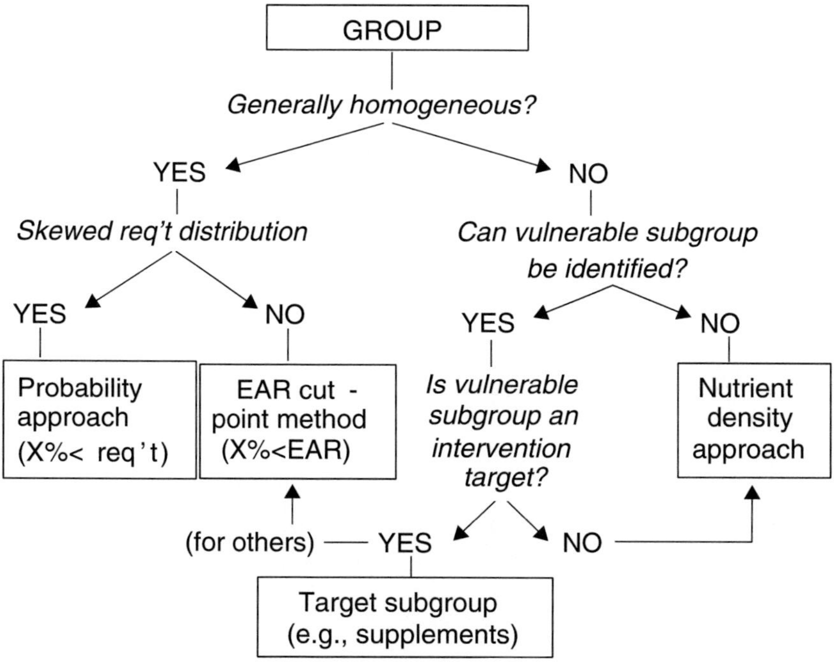

FIGURE 11-5 Decision tree for use when planning intakes for groups.
NOTE: EAR = Estimated Average Requirement.

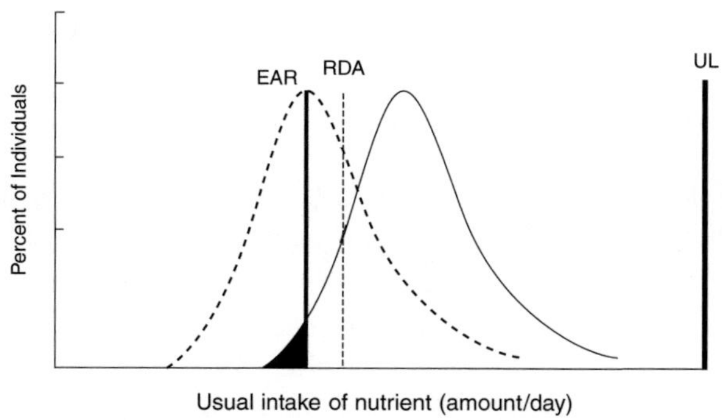

FIGURE 11-6 A comparison between the baseline and target usual intake distribution.
NOTE: dashed line = baseline usual intake distribution and solid line = the target usual intake distribution.

Research Recommendations and Progress

Because this fairly complex paradigm is largely theoretical, a number of research recommendations arose in different categories.

Recommendations Related to Intake Distributions

Determine usual intake distributions of specific population groups. At the time the subcommittee was preparing the report, it was necessary to commission special analyses to obtain data about usual intake distributions (i.e., intake distributions from which within-person variability had been removed). Considerable progress has been made toward conducting such analyses. For example, the most recent publication of *What We Eat in America* (Moshfegh et al., 2005) presents data on usual intake distributions by age and sex. In addition, several of the Canadian provincial surveys present their data in this way, and Dr. Barr anticipates that the 2004 Canadian National Survey will also present data on adjusted usual intake distributions (Health Canada, 2006).

Recommendations Related to the Planning Process Itself

A number of recommendations were related to the goal of shifting nutrient intake distributions to achieve a low prevalence of inadequacy and a low prevalence of excessive intake.

- *Pilot test the proposed approach to planning for a low group prevalence of inadequacy.* Progress towards this goal has been limited. Can the intake goals be achieved while meeting other important goals such as avoiding excess energy intakes, maintaining nutrient intakes below the upper level, and avoiding unnecessary food waste? The Institute of Medicine (IOM) Committee to Revise the WIC[4] Food Packages attempted to use the model in preparing recommendations for its report and found the approach to be quite challenging to implement for that purpose (IOM, 2006c).

---

[4]WIC stands for the USDA's Special Supplemental Nutrition Program for Women, Infants, and Children.

- *Determine the relationship between foods* offered *and the nutrient* intake *in the context of group planning.* If one offered more vitamin A-rich foods to a group that had a high prevalence of inadequate vitamin A intakes, for example, would the prevalence of inadequacy decrease? Such a decrease would only occur if the vitamin-A rich foods were actually consumed by those with inadequate intakes. Little progress has been made in systematically examining this relationship. Although some insight might be gained from the impact of food fortification programs such as the mandatory fortification of enriched cereal products with folic acid, that example does not really address what happens when the specific foods offered to groups are changed.
- *Determine how different nutrition interventions affect nutrient intake distributions.* For example, will the distribution simply shift and otherwise retain the same shape? Compared with changes in education, supplementation, or food availability, would changes in fortification have a different impact on the shape of the distribution? Other than the example of folic acid fortification, data are not available regarding the effect of different types of nutrition interventions on intake distributions. It is possible, however, that future implementation of a new WIC food package may provide some insight on what happens when food availability is changed.
- *Develop and evaluate dietary planning strategies for heterogeneous groups.* The DRI Planning Subcommittee proposed a nutrient density approach to plan for heterogeneous groups. Although one can envision how such an approach could be used to formulate a standard emergency relief ration that would meet the nutrient requirements, even of those with low energy needs, it is much more difficult to envision how this could be accomplished when a variety of foods differing in energy and nutrient content is available. No progress appears to have been made in this area.

Recommendations Related to Implementation of the Planning Process

Several recommendations address how one takes the information on nutrient requirement distributions and translates it to food-based patterns that would achieve the desired nutrient intake patterns.

- *Review and, where necessary, revise existing food guides.* The USDA has released a revised food guide called MyPyramid (USDA, 2005). It incorporates recommended intakes from the DRI reports. In general, persons who follow MyPyramid would be expected to meet the RDA or AI for most or all nutrients.
- *Develop food guides for group planning.* Canada is using an innovative modeling approach to develop a food guide that (if followed) would result in a low prevalence of diets with inadequate nutrient intakes. It could thus be used to plan diets both for groups and for individuals.
- *Assess the application of the DRIs for food and supplement labeling.* Points to consider are the updating of values, synthetic sources of nutrients, and information on the UL. *Dietary Reference Intakes: Guiding Principles for Nutrition Labeling and Fortification* (IOM, 2003b) addressed these topics. That report contains a recommendation to use a weighted EAR as the Daily Value, and this recommendation has engendered considerable debate. The Food and Drug Administration has not yet published a proposed rule on the topic.
- *Communicate with and educate nutritional professionals about correct uses of the DRIs.* Although much remains to be done to meet this goal, some progress has been made. For example, an online course on DRIs developed in Canada[5] is available, and several articles have been published in scientific journals addressing how to use the DRIs in assessment and planning. Notably, *Dietary Reference Intakes: The Essential Guide to Nutrient Requirements* (IOM, 2006a), a single-volume summary of the DRI series is likely to be a widely read and useful resource.

In conclusion, some real progress has occurred, but many critical knowledge gaps need to be bridged to be able to plan confidently for low prevalences of inadequacy and excess using the DRIs.

---

[5]The website is www.dieteticsatwork.com. A fee is charged.

DISCUSSION OF RESEARCH RECOMMENDATIONS FROM THE APPLICATION REPORTS

Presenter: Jay Hirschman

This presentation was from the position of one who works with the U.S. federal food assistance programs—food stamps; school lunch; the Supplemental Nutrition Program for Women, Infants, and Children (WIC); and many others—and thus focuses mainly on the DRI Planning Report (IOM, 2003a). Points covered included a planning conundrum, the use of end points, statistical adjustment, testing the group planning methodology, and the shape of the target intake distribution.

The Planning Conundrum

Federal food programs work mainly with heterogeneous groups. The DRI Planning Report suggests using a target usual nutrient distribution by selecting a target percent inadequate. An example given is 2.5 percent inadequate—the estimated percentage of individuals who would not be covered by meeting the RDA.

Because most of the EARs and AIs for children are determined indirectly, they involve a higher degree of uncertainty than the values for adults. Notably, approximately 50 million children in the United States attend schools that participate in the National School Lunch Program, and one should never expect the U.S. federal government to say that it is satisfactory for 2.5 percent of schoolchildren to be inadequate in a nutrient. That would translate to 1.25 million children. These factors make application of the recommended DRI planning methodology difficult in practice.

End Points

The methods of determining end points differ across the different nutrients, and the science varies enormously across the range of nutrients. However, the DRI Planning Report provides no guidance on the relative importance of reducing the percent inadequate across the different nutrients. That is, would it be better to use the same target percent inadequate for all the nutrients or, for example, to target 1 percent inadequate for one nutrient and 10 percent inadequate for another? Would the result be satisfactory if using a specific target pushed a portion of the distribution into the UL range? Those responsible for applying the methodology are left with considerable uncertainty as they make decisions about program operation on a day-to-day basis.

Statistical Adjustment Question

Mr. Hirschman raised the statistical question, Does the statistical correction based on 2 days' data correct for the intraindividual variation equally across nutrients? Basiotis and coworkers (1987) demonstrated that the number of days required for a true group average estimate of nutrient intake varies considerably across the nutrients. If the correction is not equal, this could have important implications for planning. During the discussion period, Dr. Kevin W. Dodd, a statistician at NCI, explained that the adjustment applies equally across the nutrients.

Testing the Group Planning Methodology

Mr. Hirschman has used a number of different data sets and the nutrients vitamin C and zinc to test the nutrient density approach to planning for heterogeneous groups—adolescents in particular. Figure 11-7 illustrates some of Mr. Hirschman's findings. Nutrient density per 1,000 kcals was calculated using the following formula:

$$\text{Nutrient density} = \frac{\text{mean nutrient intake}}{\text{mean energy intake}} \times 1{,}000$$

The first two bars in the figure used the 1989 RDAs for vitamin C and the average energy allowance at median height and weight rather than intake. The next two bars, which used the 2000 RDA and the estimated energy expenditure for sedentary adolescents, show a considerably larger target nutrient density. (The RDA for vitamin C had increased and the energy value, which is in the denominator, had decreased). The School Nutrition Dietary Assessment (SNDA) Studies are nationally representative studies of U.S. children attending schools offering the National School Lunch Program.

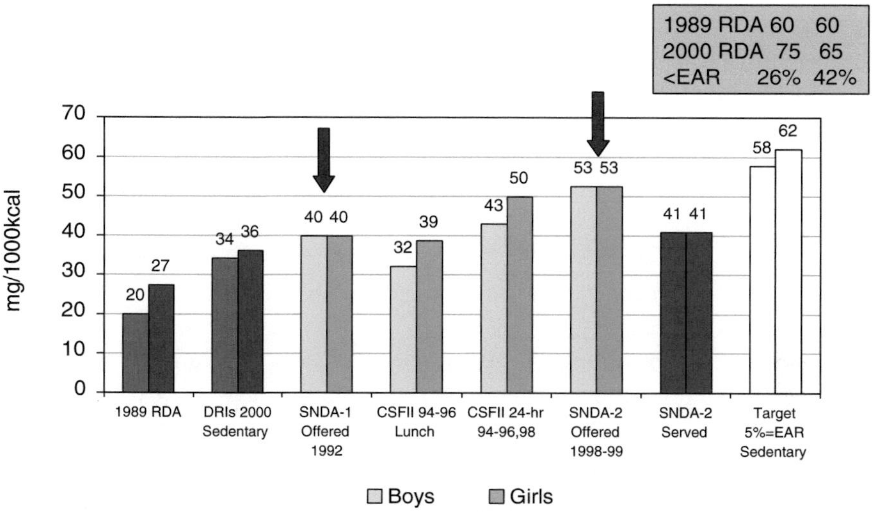

FIGURE 11-7 Vitamin C nutrient density: a comparison of survey results for adolescents. All values include vitamin pill supplements.
NOTE: RDA = Recommended Dietary Allowance, DRI = Dietary Reference Intake, EAR = Estimated Average Requirement, SNDA = School Nutrition Dietary Assessment Study, CSFII = Continuing Survey of Food Intake by Individuals. The 2000 DRI value shown is an RDA. Median values are not readily available. These are approximations based on [(mean intake/mean energy) x 1,000]

The first arrow shows vitamin C density—approximately 40 mg of vitamin C/1,000 kcal—of the food *offered* to the children in 1992. The estimated vitamin C density of food reported to be *consumed* at lunch, which is from an analysis of data from the 1994–1996 Continuing Survey of Food Intake by Individuals, is somewhat lower. Data from SNDA-2, 1998–1999, (see the second arrow in Figure 11-7) indicates that the nutrient density for vitamin C in foods *offered* was considerably higher than that reported by SNDA-1. In the interim, the USDA had implemented the School Meals Initiative for Healthy Children—a national effort to try to improve the quality of school meals.

These data show that it is functionally possible to increase nutrient density in the meals that are *offered* to children. However, the figure also shows that the vitamin C density of the meals *served* is substantially lower than that offered, meaning that the students did not take all the offerings, and they selected foods with lower than average vitamin C per

1,000 kcal. The last two bars in the figure show what the vitamin C density targets would be. For a heterogeneous population, one would use the higher nutrient density—namely 62 mg of vitamin C/1,000 kcal.

More information will become available from the analysis of SNDA-3 data from school year 2004–2005, which included (in addition to data on foods offered and foods served), data on what the children ate—both at the meals at school and over 24 hours.

Shape of the Target Intake Distribution

Government programs frequently aim to shift the shape of the distribution, as by providing larger benefits to families with lower income. This raises the research question, What assumptions should be made in planning regarding changes in the shape of the intake distribution?

Concluding Remarks

In his concluding remarks, Mr. Hirschman made the following points regarding research needs:

- Consider a coordinated research effort to review the existing mammalian animal studies, and then design and complete new mammalian studies that will improve the estimate of the variation, being sure to select species with natural variation. Also these studies should be used to improve the methods for extrapolating from adult values to other groups, especially children.
- Given that it is difficult to select the target percent inadequate, the shape of the distribution is intended to change, the end points are variable, and there is uncertainty in the intake estimates, consider the need for a new study and publication with a title that might be along the lines of *Applications of the DRIs in Planning: Health and Statistical Considerations in Selecting Targets for the Percent Inadequate Across Nutrients*.

RESEARCH RECOMMENDATIONS FOR DRI APPLICATIONS

Presenter: Patricia M. Guenther

This presentation highlighted applications of the DRIs at the USDA Center for Nutrition Policy and Promotion (CNPP), especially related to the following:

- *Dietary Guidelines for Americans 2005* (DHHS/USDA, 2005), the nutrition policy of the U.S. federal government, the development of which considered assessment of the proportion of the population with inadequate intakes of nutrients
- MyPyramid, the USDA's major consumer education tool, which uses the RDAs and AIs as the nutrient adequacy goals
- The USDA food plans, including the Thrifty Food Plan (which provides the basis of the Food Stamp Program allotments)

The purposes of the presentation were to report on the progress made regarding the research recommendations in the two DRI applications reports and to identify the research needs that remain unmet.

Progress Made Related to Assessment

A summary of progress related to assessment is presented below.

- *Reporting estimates of usual or long-run average daily intakes when assessing nutrient adequacy.* A major milestone was reached when the USDA's Agricultural Research Service used the method and software developed at Iowa State University (ISU) to estimate the proportions of the population having usual intakes below their EARs and the standard errors of these estimates (Moshfegh et al., 2005).
- *Estimating usual intake—developing more applications and greater efficiency.* NCI has developed a method for estimating usual intake that builds on previous work. It was developed for estimating population distributions of usual intakes of episodically consumed foods. Papers describing the method—by Dodd

et al., Subar et al., and Tooze et al.—are scheduled to appear in the October 2006 issue of *The Journal of the American Dietetic Association*. The NCI method is expected to work for nutrients as well as for foods. It could be used to determine whether the prevalence of inadequacy differs between two groups and whether it would be more efficient than the ISU method for that purpose.

Using models that relate intake to a health outcome within the context of the 2003–2004 National Health and Nutrition Examination Survey (NHANES), the NCI method also can predict an individual's usual intake and its standard error using appropriate covariates. The National Center for Health Statistics (NCHS) Data Users' conference in July 2006 had a session about this; and further information, SAS macros, and a web tutorial will be forthcoming through the NCHS website.

- *Developing estimates of an individual's usual intake in a clinical setting for the purposes of determining the probability of inadequate intakes.* This remains a research need. The NCI group believes that this can be done and that a confidence interval for the predicted usual intake could be estimated. This approach may prove to be more useful than the confidence-of-adequacy approach described in the DRI Assessment Report. The CNPP has found that that the confidence-of-adequacy approach is impractical for use with consumers.
- *Understanding the underreporting of food intake.* Tooze and colleagues (2004) describe results of a multivariate exploration of the underreporting of food intake and a review of earlier work done to address this topic.
- *Biomarkers.* Progress has been made in the use of recovery biomarkers such as doubly labeled water and urinary nitrogen to estimate bias in dietary assessments. Progress has also occurred in the use of concentration biomarkers (e.g., serum carotenoids, which are correlated with nutrient intake). However, consensus has not yet been reached regarding the usefulness of concentration biomarkers.
- *Measuring the intake of supplements.* The plans for the NHANES 2007–2008 include collecting 2 days of supplement and dietary intake data, which will facilitate the estimation of

day-to-day variability in nutrient intake from supplements and total nutrient intake.

- *Qualitative consumer-oriented research on how to communicate concepts related to assessing dietary adequacy, the most important one being probability of adequacy.* This remains a research need. The CNPP needs some exploratory research to find out what consumers want to know about dietary adequacy and what will be meaningful to them. Dietitians need consumer research-based advice about how to explain dietary adequacy information to their clients.

Progress Made Related to Planning

The CNPP uses the RDAs and AIs in the development of its food guidance system, (MyPyramid), which provides plans for use by individuals. Dr. Guenther concurred with previous speakers that a well-conceived and tested nutrient density approach to the DRIs could facilitate the planning of diets for families whose members have heterogeneous nutrient needs. The CNPP will be using a nutrient density approach in its dietary assessment tool. The revised Healthy Eating Index will assess food intakes per 1,000 calories of energy intake.

Potential New Research Questions

The following two topics of interest to the CNPP might be considered for future research:

1. Noting that the AMDRs are density standards, the CNPP would find it very helpful if more of the DRIs could be expressed on a density basis, such as per 1,000 calories of energy intake or per kilogram of body weight.
2. A recommended ratio of sodium to potassium intake could also be useful. The protective effect of potassium-rich diets in blunting the adverse effects of sodium intake has not yet been quantified to the extent that it could be used in dietary guidance and assessment. Given the difficulty of planning higher calorie diets that do not exceed the AI for sodium, a research-based rec-

ommendation that simultaneously considers both sodium and potassium intake would be most welcome.

Summary

Progress in applying the DRIs has been demonstrated by the use of the ISU method and software to estimate the prevalence of inadequacy, the development of the NCI method for further applications of usual intake, advances in biomarkers, and plans for improved collection of information on supplement use. The remaining research needs are methods for estimating individual usual intake, consumer communication research, and expanding the research base for the development of DRIs that can be expressed as densities or ratios.

EDUCATING PROFESSIONALS ON THE USE OF DIETARY REFERENCE INTAKES

Presenter: Rena Mendelson

This presentation briefly covered topics related to communicating about the DRIs from the perspective of an individual who teaches undergraduate dietetic students and who needs to explain the DRIs to young college students. Then, very brief mention was made concerning application of the DRIs from the perspective of work with the Ontario Food Survey in Canada.

Students, other professionals, consumers, and others basically want to know if they are deficient in any nutrients and, if they are deficient, what they should do to make up for the deficiency. Dr. Mendelson finds that textbooks pose a problem. The most popular textbooks tend to include the RDAs but not the EARs. Textbooks come with nutritional analysis software, but students have difficulty determining whether they have made a mistake or not. Two major reasons for this difficulty are the students' lack of knowledge of food composition data and lack of experience with hand analyses of nutrient intake. Moreover, the target to which intake is compared varies in different software packages and may not be clearly identified.

Explaining the probability of inadequacy to a student who is looking for a deficiency poses a challenge. Having them do the analysis for their intake by hand is a tedious process, but doing one's own analysis helps with comprehension.

Dr. Mendelson considers it important to examine how dietitians are using the DRIs in conjunction with dietary data. Pertinent questions include, How are they analyzing and interpreting the information? and How are the many other providers of nutrition advice using the information? She concurred with Dr. Guenther's recommendation concerning research on communicating with consumers.

Using the DRIs in conjunction with survey data may pose other challenges. After applying the cut-point method to look at the estimated prevalence of inadequacy in the population, interpreting and acting on the findings requires careful consideration. For example, what action is needed, if any, in view of the finding that 35 percent of the population has an estimated prevalence of inadequacy of magnesium?

DISCUSSION

Topics covered during the discussion included supplements, nutrient density, software, and the DRI paradigm. For comments on the DRI paradigm, see the "Discussion" section in Chapter 13.

Vitamin-Mineral Supplements

Dr. Dwyer commented that supplements and fortified foods are sometimes overlooked in dietary planning. Several discussants responded, giving examples pertaining to dietary assessment. Food surveys provide data about fortified foods but not necessarily about supplements. Dr. Hirschman pointed out that targets for children are based on nutrients from foods and that the conservative approach is to examine intake from foods only unless there is a concern with exceeding the UL. Drs. Mendelson and Barr commented that the estimated prevalence of inadequacy with supplement use was essentially the same as that without supplement use in one Canadian survey, but it was lower in another one. Method of data collection, region of the country, and year all may have contributed to the difference in the findings.

Nutrient Density

Dr. Bier noted that there is no standard definition of nutrient density and that we lack a way to compare the nutrient density if, for example, one food is rich in vitamin E and another in vitamin C. Is it correct to use calories as the denominator? Dr. Barr clarified that, in the DRI Planning Report, nutrient density was considered nutrient by nutrient. One examines the distribution of the nutrient requirement in relation to the distribution of the energy requirement. She noted that no method was developed to combine the densities for different nutrients.

Software

In response to Dr. Dwyer's question regarding availability of quality software, Dr. Mendelson suggested that software companies link up with publishers of widely distributed textbooks and that the two parties synchronize their approach to computerized dietary assessments.

12

New and Underutilized Research Techniques and the Dietary Reference Intakes[1]

Looking to the future in terms of Dietary Reference Intakes (DRI) efforts brings a need to consider new techniques, new methodologies, and new research opportunities. This session included three perspectives on new and underutilized research techniques that may be applicable to DRIs. Irwin H. Rosenberg of Tufts University, who served as a member of the Subcommittee on Upper Reference Levels of Nutrients, addressed promising research techniques and a research strategy for setting Tolerable Upper Intake Levels (ULs). Paul B. Pencharz of the University of Toronto, who served on the macronutrient panel, focused on protein and amino acid research. Jose M. Ordovas of Tufts University addressed the "-omics" and systems biology.

NEW AND UNDERUTILIZED RESEARCH TECHNIQUES AND THE DIETARY REFERENCE INTAKES

Presenter: Irwin H. Rosenberg

The presentation covered potential research techniques and also some major research needs that could be addressed with more traditional techniques.

[1]This chapter is based on a transcript and slides from the workshop.

Promising Research Techniques

Genotyping, Epigenetics, and Imprinting

Topics that need consideration with regard to setting nutrient requirements and to considering susceptibility to higher levels of intake of a nutrient include genotyping, epigenetics, and imprinting—including the assessment of effects of single nucleotide polymorphisms (SNPs) on variability in requirements and/or ULs. Earlier in this workshop, Drs. Steven Zeisel and Patrick Stover provided examples, such as the finding that methylation of deoxyribonucleic acid (DNA) at the cytosine position can have a substantial influence on gene expression and that dietary methyl donors can influence the level of methylation to some extent. This is a knowledge area that is important to understand, particularly when it is possible that one can influence not only gene expression but even the total silencing of a gene, resulting in genetic imprinting and some very important phenotypic outcomes. Some interesting modeling challenges can be anticipated.

With regard to the methylene tetrahydrofolate reductase (MTHFR) polymorphisms, the pathway is highly complex; flavin-adenine dinucleotide (FAD) may be able to partially stabilize the heat lability of the variant. Looking at this additional way in which riboflavin interacts with this pathway may serve as another example of how this type of information will enter some of the decision making related to DRIs.

A specific example involves the C677T mutation in the MTHFR gene. Homozygosity for this mutation results in a less active and a more heat-sensitive enzyme protein (Kang et al., 1988). Heat sensitivity results in dissociation of FAD, but the dissociation is prevented by folate substrates (Guenther et al., 1999). The prevalence of the homozygous variant differs among subgroups: the variant exists in about 15 percent of the Caucasian population, is less prevalent in African Americans, and is more prevalent in Hispanics.

Data from Dr. Paul Jacques of Tufts University shows an elevation of homocysteine in the homozygous variant only when folate intake is below the median. This finding raised questions about whether different subgroups would respond differently to intake. The increase in plasma folate by genotype (data provided by Jacques, see Figure 12-1), suggests that the abnormality probably is not a large determinant of the requirement. One possible model of the MTHFR variant related to the folate requirement is depicted in Figure 12-2. This model assumes that the variant represents a certain part of the distribution of the folate requirement that would shift the curve only slightly to the right. The intent of this model is to illustrate that when new data are obtained, models will be needed to help interpret how findings about requirements of subpopulations should influence requirements set for the overall population.

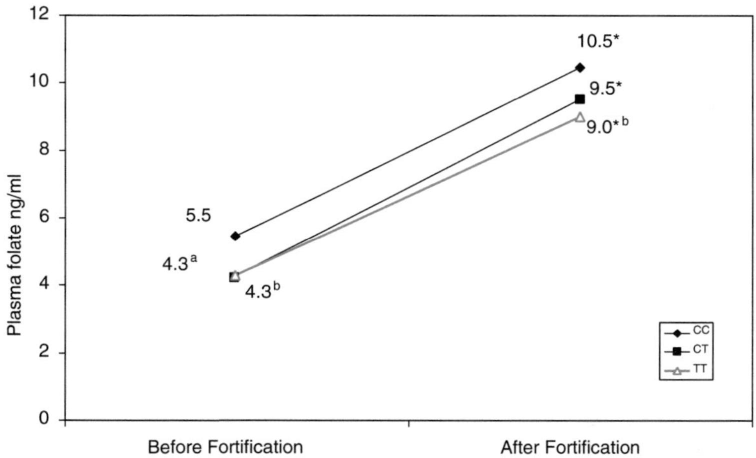

FIGURE 12-1 Increase in plasma folate by genotype.
*p < .05 compared with the same genotype before fortification.
[a]p < .05 compared to wild type.
[b]p < .05 compared to wild type. Significance lost after adjustment for multiple comparisons.
SOURCE: Paul Jacques, Tufts University, Boston.

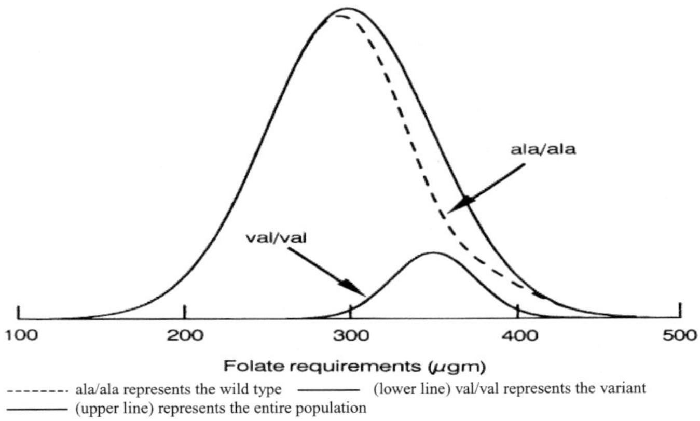

FIGURE 12-2 A possible model of the MTHFR variant related to the folate requirement.
NOTE: Dashed line (ala/ala) represents the wild type; lower line (val/val) represents the variant; upper line represents the entire population.
SOURCE: Irwin Rosenberg, Tufts University, Boston, MA.

Bioavailability Studies

Because nutrition deals with different forms of vitamins and minerals, studies of bioavailability are very important. Dr. Rosenberg views them as absolutely essential in the setting of requirements.

An example is provided by folate, dietary folate equivalents, and folic acid. One of the research recommendations made in the DRI B Vitamins Report (IOM, 1998a) is to obtain more information about monoglutamate versus food folate, which Dr. Rosenberg views as an oversimplification. Instead, he suggested that the research need concerns free folic acid versus folates embedded in foods. The hydrolysis of folate polyglutamates is not the rate-limiting problem in folate absorption. Probably absorption is affected by the release of folate from some of the food matrices. Whether folic acid (the synthetic form of the vitamin) is given with or without food may affect its bioavailability.

Dr. Rosenberg then pointed out that the DRI B Vitamins Report (IOM, 1998a) misapplies dietary folate equivalents to the folate contained in human milk. Doing so is inappropriate because human milk folate is absorbed by a totally different process than is folate provided by other foods. In particular, the infant absorbs the folate from breast milk in association with a protein binder that passes across a permeable membrane. As a result, the folate in human milk probably is at least as well—if not better—absorbed than is folic acid—the form of the vitamin added to infant formula. Expressing human milk folate in terms of dietary folate equivalents underestimates the bioavailable folate content of human milk and thus the Adequate Intake (AI). This error in the report needs to be corrected.

Stable Isotope Studies

Fruitful areas for research involving stable isotope studies (the subject of other presentations during this workshop) include the conversion of carotenes to vitamin A, studies of amino acid and protein requirements, and doubly labeled water studies.

Research Strategy for Setting ULs

The report of the Upper Levels Subcommittee (IOM, 1998b) did not contain a set of research recommendations, in spite of the fact that the research needs were very great. Of the research recommendations contained in the set of DRI reports, only 2 of 60 in the research methods list refer to the ULs. A few more could be attributed to UL research needs. A look at the complete list of research needs reveals an even lower proportion of needs that apply to ULs.

Dr. Rosenberg called for a commitment to the research base for making the judgments needed to set ULs, including the following:

- Sharper end points of adverse effects
- Dose–response analyses with larger numbers—a very important need for ULs and EARs
- Depletion–repletion studies for adverse effects if feasible and ethical (otherwise, consider ways to obtain better information from cohort studies)
- Validated surrogate markers of risk

An early finding, such as the presence of esterified vitamin A as evidence of replete stores, might be one example of a surrogate marker of risk. Another possible surrogate marker might be circulating free folic acid, which indicates that doses of folic acid beyond the ability of dihydrofolate reductase to reduce them have entered the metabolic system. Connecting various observations with other functional markers and functions may help move the process forward.

Dr. Rosenberg concluded that the process for setting ULs is relatively new. Progress in this area will require a commitment to the research that allows making good judgments.

A FOCUS ON PROTEIN AND AMINO ACIDS

Presenter: Paul B. Pencharz

Promising Future Directions for Research

In looking at future directions for research related to the DRIs, this presentation highlighted the following points:

- Know where we come from—that is, return to first principles and rediscover what people previously knew. For example, in about 1900, Karl Voit reported that 1 gram of protein per kilogram of body weight per day supported good work efficiency.
- Consider the techniques used to determine the dietary requirements of monogastric farm animals (e.g., pigs), because the animals are easier to study and exhibit less genetic variability.
- Find surrogate measures that can be used to determine dose–response to define a level to use in studying longer-term functional outcomes.

Dr. Pencharz clarified that his remarks were from the perspective of a researcher who is interested in minimally invasive methods that can be used in children.

Using the Full Range of Intakes to Define the DRI Values

In the DRI process, the Estimated Average Requirement (EAR) is best established by defining the physiological response both below and above the requirement point. This approach also helps define variability and thus the Recommended Dietary Allowance (RDA). The use of nonlinear regression and two-phase linear cross-over regression analysis could be helpful in defining the variability.

Using piglets as subjects, a feeding study could be helpful in identifying a surrogate measure that would indicate that a particular amino acid is potentially toxic (e.g., that it can no longer be metabolized if intake exceeds a certain amount). In a study that fed higher and higher levels of phenylalanine, the data curve showed a point at which the data went straight up—that is, it identified the phenylalanine intake at which phenylalanine hydroxylase is overwhelmed. The break point could serve as a surrogate measure that the particular amino acid could be toxic.

Methods Related to the EAR for Protein

Dr. Pencharz discussed the following views regarding methods related to protein requirements:

- Nitrogen balance is a cumbersome tool and is expensive and time consuming.
- Failure to include all available data in past analyses may have resulted in an underestimation of protein requirements.
- Longer-term feeding studies are needed (e.g., Garza et al. [1977] provided evidence that short-term nitrogen balance studies probably underestimate the protein requirement).
- New methods need to be applied. Preliminary data obtained by measuring breath $^{13}CO_2$ following the oxidation of orally administered L-[1-^{13}C] phenylalanine over various protein intakes suggest that the break point for the protein requirement occurs at about 0.9 g/kg of body weight, which is consistent with a reanalysis of nitrogen balance data.

Methods for determining amino acid requirements include growth, which is useful only during rapid growth; nitrogen balance; direct oxidation; indicator amino acid oxidation (IAAO); 24-hour direct amino acid balance; and 24-hour indicator amino acid balance (IAAB). Either the indicator of oxidation or the 24-hour balance is currently considered the state of the art for determining amino acid requirements.

Genetic variability merits consideration as related to research on protein requirements. Within-subject variability is smaller than between-subject variability. Farm animals with selective breeding have much less variability than humans, but ongoing studies in dogs of different breeds are showing a degree of variability that is similar to that in humans.

The IAAO could be used as a direct reflection of protein synthesis for two purposes: (1) comparing a commercially available parenteral amino acid solution to a new parenteral solution, and (2) identifying limiting amino acids in both parenteral solutions. A corollary with food could be to determine how processing alters the bioavailability of an amino acid. Within one day, this method can identify the limiting amino acids.

Concluding Remarks

In conclusion, there is a need to relate the determination of DRIs to long-term health. Determine whether short-term balance studies relate to long-term health. Conduct studies with graded levels of intake to define an appropriate intake level, and then study health effects of that intake over a long term, as was done by Garza and colleagues (1977). Consider additional ways to examine function—possibly the Harvard Step Test as a measure of iron status. Look at findings in new ways, for example, How do studies that show a suppression of parathyroid concentration with increased 25-hydroxyvitamin D relate to bone health and hence to vitamin D requirements? Would the answer require long-term studies or would medium- or short-term studies suffice?

"-OMICS" AND SYSTEMS BIOLOGY

Presenter: Jose M. Ordovas

The focus of this presentation was how the science of genetics can be used to reduce the risk of chronic disease, with examples mainly related to reducing the risk of coronary heart disease. In response to research recommendation 8-A,[2] genetics can be very helpful in determining the individual risk for chronic or age-related diseases. Genetics may help predict, as early as possible, those people who will be more susceptible to common disorders, so that specific attention can be directed to them. Earlier detection of diabetes mellitus, for example, could have an enormous impact: using current methods, persons with diabetes already have lost about 50 percent of their beta-cell function by the time the diabetes is diagnosed.

What is involved in this earlier detection? It requires capturing and interpreting information at different levels and using a variety of novel techniques. Thus, *genomics* involves studying the genomes, which contain the information (an indication of what can happen). *Transcriptomics* is used to analyze gene expression (what appears to be happening). *Proteomics* is used to investigate proteins (compounds that make things happen). *Metabolomics* is used measure metabolites (substances that indicate what has happened and is happening).

Genetic information provided by the Framingham Study (Lahoz et al., 2001) shows a differential cardiovascular disease (CVD) risk associated with the presence of one or another allele at candidate genes (i.e., *APOE*) and a gender difference as well. Genetics may help provide more specific information related to the need for different recommendations for men and women, and provide such information early. In one example, genetics could identify 12 or 15 percent of the population who would not be identified by low-density lipoprotein (LDL) cholesterol, the classical biomarker for CVD risk. Their LDL cholesterol could be low despite a genetic predisposition to have as much cardiovascular disease risk as do those with high LDL cholesterol.

Because the technology has moved forward, an approach called unbiased knowledge acquisition is examining the genome and obtaining data on hundreds of thousands of SNPs. A National Institutes of Health initiative is working to put all this information in the public domain. In the near future, the entire human genome variation will be covered, allowing investigation of genes of interest in terms of whatever pathway is being studied.

---

[2]See Appendix C to find the wording that corresponds to the recommendation numbers given in this chapter. The number refers to the ID number for the recommendation in the DRI Research Synthesis Database, and the letter refers to the specific DRI report.

Possible Revisions of Selected Research Recommendations

Dr. Ordovas suggested a revision of research recommendation 282-E related to genetic variants that contribute to the intraindividual variation in LDL. In particular, he added high-density lipoprotein cholesterol (HDL-C) and triglyceride concentrations as biomarkers of interest and fatty acids as a dietary component.

In addition to the traditional CVD risk biomarkers (usually measured in the fasting state), increasing evidence supports the notion that biomarkers measured in the nonfasting (postprandial) state may have a key role in identifying CVD risk. Many, many genes are involved in the complex postprandial process of handling dietary fat and cholesterol. Thus, genes may affect the concentration of atherogenic triglyceride-rich lipoproteins, and CVD risk varies with the concentration of these lipoproteins during the postprandial period. For example, research at one of the candidate genes examined (*APOA5*) shows that for the people who do not have a specific polymorphism—approximately 80 to 85 percent of the U.S. population—polyunsaturated fatty acid intake has little effect on this risk factor. However, for those who are carriers of the polymorphism, circulating triglyceride-rich lipoprotein concentrations tend to be higher; and this condition is associated with greater CVD risk. This negative aspect of this gene variant is expressed only in the case of higher *n*-6 polyunsaturated fatty acid intake.

Dr. Ordovas also suggested revising research recommendation 256-E relating to dose–response studies by adding *n*-6 and *n*-3 polyunsaturated fatty acids to the examples of essential macronutrients. The negative effect associated with the higher intake of polyunsaturated fatty acids (discussed in the previous paragraph) is exclusive to *n*-6 fatty acids.

With regard to research recommendation 266-E, genetics might be used, for example, to predict who is going to benefit from the classical approaches to successful or lasting weight loss. Figure 12-4 shows a 12-month follow-up of obese subjects who were placed on hypocaloric diets (Corella et al., 2005). The carriers of the allele of the perilipin gene did not lose weight during the year, whereas the group without the polymorphism did. (The perilipin gene is expressed in the adipocytes and protects the adipocytes from lipolysis.) Thus, this is an example of how to distinguish the people who may be able to succeed with a traditional weight-reduction approach from those who need a different intervention.

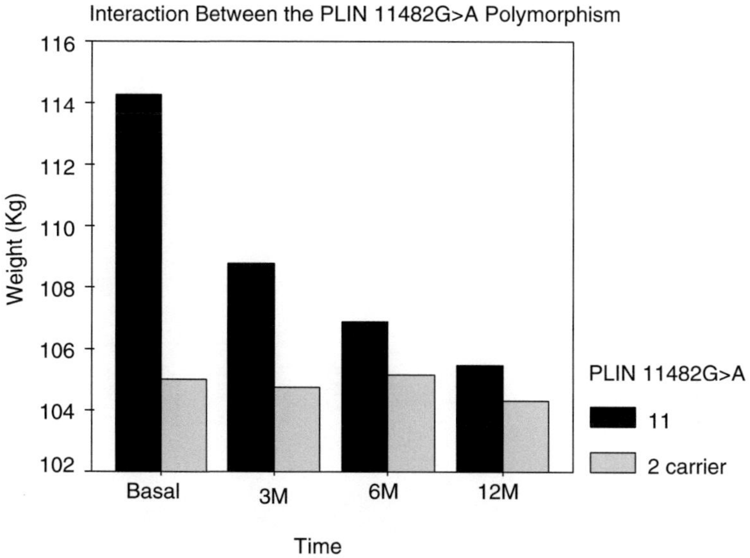

FIGURE 12-4 Weight reduction over 1 year (obese subjects on a low-calorie diet), by PLIN (11482G > A) polymorphism status.
NOTE : M = month.
SOURCE: From Corella et al. (2005). Obese subjects carrying the 11482G>A polymorphism at the perilipin locus are resistant to weight loss after dietary energy restriction. *J Clin Endocrinol Metab*. 90(9):5121–5126. *Copyright 2005, The Endocrine Society.*

Making Use of Metabolomics

Metabolomics can be used to distinguish people who have severe atherosclerosis from those who have normal coronary arteries (see Figure 12-5).The partial least squares for discriminant analysis (PLS-DA) model (Brindle et al., 2002) is a noninvasive, multivariate statistical approach to predicting coronary artery status that makes catheterization (a very invasive process) unnecessary. A yet unpublished example of a metabolomic technique combines ultraperformance linkage chromatography with mass spectrometry. The technique produces PLS-DA score plots for three different diets, which allows identification of the dietary phase (saturated fat, polyunsaturated fat, or monounsaturated fat) for each subject. In the future, this kind of approach might be used to assess compliance or the intake of certain nutrients.

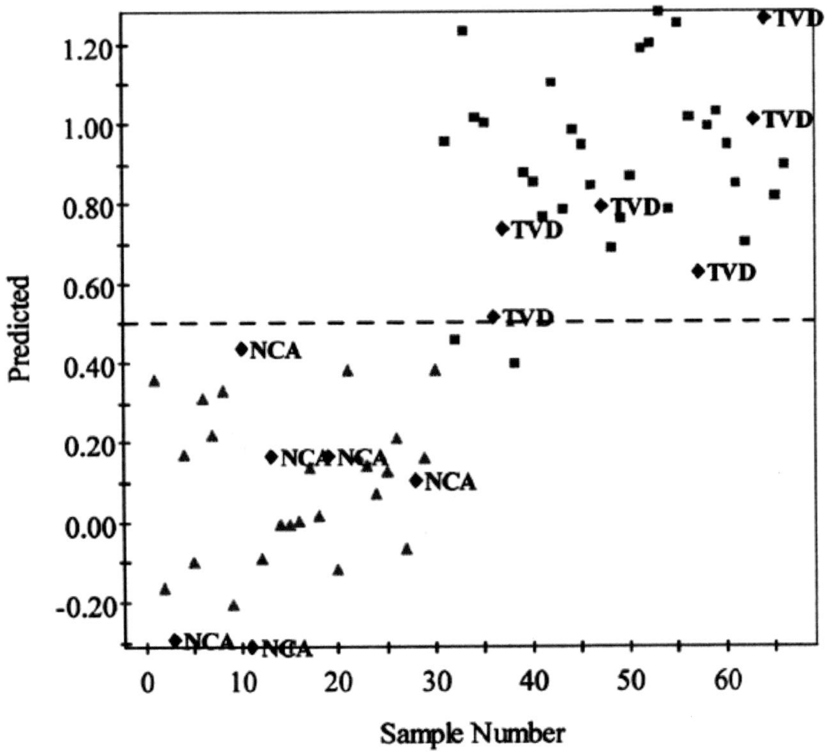

FIGURE 12-5 Prediction of coronary artery status using the PLS-DA model. Comparison of patients with severe atherosclerosis (TVD) and patients with normal coronary arteries (NCA)
SOURCE: Brindle et al. (2002). Reprinted by permission from Macmillan Publishers Ltd: Nature Medicine. *Rapid and noninvasive diagnosis of the presence and severity of coronary heart disease using 1H-NMR-based metabonomics.* 8:1439–1445. Copyright 2002.

Because of the huge amount of information that is being generated by these new techniques, it is important to use bioinformatics to process the information and make it readily usable. By using this approach and the different connections between genes and gene products, it will be possible to define, for example, the mechanisms by which arachidonic acid and docahexaenoic acid (DHA) inhibit the synthesis and production of cholesterol. By knowing the key players along pathways, it will be possible to increase the points at which specific nutrients can be targeted for disease prevention and even treatment.

Concluding Remarks

Dr. Ordovas concluded that the ultimate goal of nutrigenomics is determining optimal nutrition for everyone—not just for 95 percent—with any genetic constitution, in any environment, at any life stage. He predicts that what is called nutrigenomics today will be called nutrition within the next 10 years.

DISCUSSION

Dr. Zeisel commented that a parallel use of metabolomics can be developed to analyze food composition. The concept is to look at the 3,000 components in a food and characterize them simultaneously. Thus, the investment in metabolomics could help both the clinical studies and the food composition studies.

In response to Dr. Pencharz's comments on variability, Dr. Appel noted that the DRI reports tended not to deal with measurement error issues related to intraindividual variability, and he asked for a research objective to document the variation and to catalogue it in future reports.

Dr. Rosenberg commented that despite all the power of genomics, he does not expect to be able to explain individual variation only in those terms. For example, differences in absorption and even metabolic turnovers will not be completely explained by measuring these genotypes. Dr. Ordovas agreed, stating that genetics can explain up to 50 percent.

13

Wrap-Up Session

In the final session of the workshop, five speakers from a range of backgrounds presented closing remarks. John Suttie of the University of Wisconsin and chairperson of the workshop planning committee led off. He was followed by Dr. Molly Kretsch of the Agricultural Research Service (ARS) of the U.S. Department of Agriculture (USDA) and a co-chairperson of the Federal Dietary Reference Intakes (DRIs) Research Synthesis Subcommittee; Dr. Hasan Hutchinson from the Institute of Nutrition, Metabolism and Diabetes of the Canadian Institutes of Health Research; Dr. Catherine E. Woteki from Mars, Inc. and a former staff director of the Food and Nutrition Board and former chairperson of the Food and Nutrition Board; and Dr. Dennis Bier, an academic researcher from the USDA Children's Nutrition Research Center at Baylor University, Texas.

COMMENTS BY DR. SUTTIE

This presentation included a series of points that address the question, What did we learn here today?:

- Much research that related to the research recommendations has been conducted—more than some of us realized.
- In some cases, sufficient new information is available to warrant reexamination of selected DRIs in the near future.
- Some problems of the past DRI process have become apparent retrospectively and will require careful attention in the future. For example, in a number of cases the Recommended Dietary

Allowances (RDAs) and the Tolerable Upper Intake Levels (ULs) are not compatible.

- Limitations of the Adequate Intake (AI) were raised by a number of speakers. In Dr. Suttie's view, the AI is based on a concept that is useful in situations where data are insufficient to set an Estimated Average Requirement (EAR), but the usefulness of the AI has been limited by lack of a common definition. The AI was established in different ways for various nutrients, and the lack of consistency causes some problems. Over the course of 10 to 12 years, new challenges have arisen. For example, should the EARs now be based more on criteria that relate to health promotion? In many ways, the use of such criteria is much more difficult than focusing on biological assays.
- One cannot underestimate the impact that the rapid move to genomics will have on the DRI process. Within a few years, it will be relatively inexpensive for people to have their genome searched and at least a few hundred markers identified. Some of those markers will identify rather drastic changes in nutrient metabolism or in the nutrient requirement. How should this type of information be incorporated in the DRI model? How do we make sure that we cover the subpopulations that have higher requirements without moving to higher recommendations that potentially could have some undesirable effects?
- More information is available now on how the DRI process can be used for planning and how it is used by different agencies to develop different programs. Some problems have been identified that need to be addressed more explicitly than was done in the first reports.
- Recommendations for infants and children definitely need attention. Problems with extrapolations are of concern. Since the methods to study nutrient requirements in adults typically have involved invasive techniques, studies of children pose difficulties. Therefore, addressing the requirements of infants and children will require much more thought in the future. One possibility would be to have a committee address the problem of establishing requirements for infants and children across the range of nutrients.
- The difficulties in dealing with ULs need to be addressed, especially since ULs are expected to become more important in the future.

COMMENTS BY MOLLY KRETSCH

A new collaborative process between U.S. and Canadian government sponsors and with sponsors and the Institute of Medicine was initiated with this project. The U.S. Federal DRI Steering Committee is very pleased with the results of this new way of working. This presentation included a review of the goals of the project, progress made, next steps, and cross-cutting research needs.

Goals and Progress Made

Box 13-1 shows a summary of the goals and of progress made. Follow-up activities after this workshop involve the database, a report, and funding.

BOX 13-1
Goals of the DRI Research Synthesis Project and Progress Made

DRI Research Synthesis Goals	Progress Made
Identify DRI research gaps.	Excellent progress. The searchable database and workshop advanced this goal.
Collate a searchable database of the DRI research recommendations.	Second version is available for testing. Speakers identified the need for a rigorous process of formulating the research recommendations in the future.
Evaluate the current relevance of these research recommendations.	Considerable progress. Speakers provided updates on research progress and what remains to be done.
Use the information to inform the federal research planning process.	Pending. The workshop information together with input from other sources, such as stakeholders, will be used to establish agency research agendas.
Stimulate needed research to underpin future revisions of the DRIs.	Pending. Questions include: How can we increase funding for DRI research? How can we state DRI research needs in a way that researchers want to work in this area?

Next Steps

Searchable Database

The Federal DRI Steering Committee would like to see the DRI Research Synthesis Database become a "living database"—one that would encompass not only the DRI research recommendations but also the progress made toward filling these research gaps. Toward this end, new software could make it possible to link these research recommendations to the research portfolios of federal agencies. Such a linkage would make it easier to identify progress and help coordinate research in the United States—and possibly between the United States and Canada as well. At this time, resources for maintaining a "living database" have not yet been secured, but this is a possibility to be explored.

Workshop

The workshop summary should be available in October 2006. The workshop's information will help inform the research planning process for the Federal DRI Steering Committee agencies. For example, this workshop and the database are very timely for the ARS, which does considerable research on human nutrient requirements. Planning for the next 5-year research cycle for the ARS Human Nutrition Program starts in January 2007. The workshop, together with other input from stakeholders, will help inform the research planning process.

Funding

Revising the DRIs must be continued. However, some perceive that the study of nutrient requirements is simply filling gaps and is of limited importance. Thus, not only is there a need for dedicated funding, but we need to change perceptions regarding the nature and importance of this research. How can we engender interest in this field by young researchers? Thought needs to be given to how we can boost funding for and interest in future DRI research.

Cross-Cutting Research Needs

One cross-cutting research need that has been emphasized during the workshop is continued work on food and dietary supplement composition databases. Two of the speakers acknowledged clear research advances stemming from advances in food composition data, specifically with regard to choline and vitamin K. On the other hand, two other speakers indicated that research is lagging because of deficiencies in food composition data, especially for vitamins E and D. Also, the application of metabolomics methodology to food composition analyses, which was mentioned by Dr. Ordovas, has been initiated by the USDA Food Composition Laboratory at Beltsville, Maryland. Other cross-cutting research needs include methodologies for the assessment of dietary intake, physical activity, and biomarkers of exposure. All these cross-cutting research needs fall in the area of methods, and frequently this area receives limited funding.

Acknowledgments

In her closing comments, Dr. Kretsch acknowledged the efforts of the members of the Workshop Planning Committee, the Federal DRI Research Synthesis Subcommittee and its Canadian counterparts, and the federal sponsors who provided funding for this project.

COMMENTS BY HASAN HUTCHINSON

This presentation included a review of objectives for the DRI Research Synthesis, types of knowledge gaps in general and for Canada, and selected uses of the DRI Research Synthesis in Canada.

Objectives

The Canadian Institutes of Health Research's top three objectives for the DRI Research Synthesis project were essentially the same as those presented by Dr. Kretsch. In addition, it is anticipated that the project would inform future iterations of the DRIs, methods of organizing research recommendations in future reports, and the prioritizing of future research related to nutrient requirements. Certainly, prioritization is going to occur at the agency level, with consideration given to mandates and stakeholders.

Knowledge Gap Themes

Dr. Hutchinson highlighted the following knowledge gap themes:

- Requirements of children, pregnant and lactating women, and the elderly—all of which are vulnerable population groups
- Individual variation of requirements caused by genetics/epigenetics, lifestyle, environment, and geography
- The need for biomarkers that are able to predict functional outcomes and chronic diseases
- The need to improve dietary assessments and planning methods, including survey methodology and the food composition tables and databases
- Bioavailability
- Interactions among nutrients

Research gaps that are especially important in Canada include information on how geographical variables affect the vitamin D needs of Canadians, vitamin B_{12} requirements of the elderly and how they can be met (Canada has no vitamin B_{12} fortification of foods), and nutrient requirements of children—a need voiced throughout the workshop.

Uses of the Research Synthesis in Canada

The workshop and database have facilitated the identification of research needs and promising future studies. The database is expected to be a very useful tool for researchers and for planning by agencies. Health Canada uses the research gap information to address in-house research needs. Its research program primarily supports the department's policy and risk assessment work. The Canadian Institutes of Health, like the ARS in the United States, is about to enter its next planning phase. Given the importance of this type of research and its application toward policy work and risk work, Dr. Hutchinson anticipates that nutrition research relevant to the DRIs will move forward in the institutes' priorities. Dr.

Hutchinson expressed support for the idea of coordinating Canadian approaches with those of American colleagues. This might take the form of common funding calls or at least complementary funding calls in the future.

COMMENTS BY CATHERINE E. WOTEKI

This presentation reemphasized some of the points made during the introductory session to provide the context for her discussion of the DRI research recommendations. In particular, the presentation covered selected aspects of the evolution of the DRIs, key questions relative to research priorities, challenges, perspectives on funding, and responsibility for leading the research agenda.

Evolution of the DRIs

As conceived, the DRIs are an evolutionary and iterative scientific synthesis. The conceptual approach that was used for the DRIs was set out in the publication called "*How Should the Recommended Dietary Allowances Be Revised*?" (IOM, 1994). Key points from that publication are summarized as follows:

- Reference values to be included: deficient, estimated average requirement (EAR), recommended dietary allowance (RDA), and an upper safe range of intake
- Substances to be included: essential nutrients and what was called "important food components"
- The incorporation of aspects from the report *Dietary Reference Values for Food Energy and Nutrients for the United Kingdom* (COMA, 1991)

The Food and Nutrition Board sought scientific review of its conceptual report through symposia, requests for public comments, and discussions at meetings of scientific societies. The process of developing the DRIs was intended to (1) be a much more open and participatory process than previously had been the case; (2) include a more transparent exposition of the principles, scientific evidence, and derivation of the values; (3) provide more flexibility to address the many uses of the nutrient values; and (4) develop research recommendations to identify knowledge gaps.

The Food and Nutrition Board had discussed extensively how it could be possible to revise and update selected DRIs and/or other information when new research evidence showed the need for such action. As pointed out in this workshop, such revisions or updates have not occurred. This matter merits much consideration.

Key Questions Relative to Research Priorities

Based on the presentations and discussions of the DRI Research Synthesis Workshop, addressing the following key questions would help to define what the priorities should be for research to be undertaken immediately. They relate to the question: Is the DRI paradigm "right"? That is,

- Are the EAR, the RDA, the establishment of AIs and ULs the right values? Conceptually, are these values appropriate for the purposes for which they are being used or need to be used?
- Are the methods used to derive these values appropriate with respect to extrapolations and other statistical adjustments, and are they equally applicable to nutrients and to other food substances that have received little attention to date?
- Are the risk assessment approaches used to set the UL the most appropriate?
- Does the establishment of AIs and Acceptable Macronutrient Distribution Ratios (AMDRs) imply that the paradigm does not fit all nutrients?

Under the current DRI paradigm, the EAR has great importance: exposition of the end point selected is clear, data sets that were used are identified, the EAR is used in establishing the RDA, and the EAR has multiple uses in assessment and planning. This degree of importance may be greater than initially recognized.

If the DRI paradigm is correct, the research agenda priorities are clear. They relate to (1) identifying the valid nutritional status end points for nutrients that have public health importance and that lack an EAR, and (2) collecting sufficient data to set the EAR. If the paradigm is not correct, however, the same questions would remain; but there would be a different emphasis in establishing the priorities.

Challenges

Assuming that the paradigm is correct, challenges remain. Workshop presenters addressed many of them: methodological issues, studies in infants and children, and incorporating genetic polymorphisms as they relate to nutrient requirements. Additional challenges relate to aspects of evidence-based reviews that are appropriate to setting DRIs and considering important food components that have not been part of this process.

Funding the Research Agenda

Two major factors will affect funding for the nutrition research agenda: the perceived need to address other topics within the research agenda and, even more importantly, all other priorities in the agency budgets and in the federal government budgets in both the United States and Canada. Consequently, an enormous amount might be gained from coordination among the U.S. and Canadian agencies to

- establish a mechanism to set priorities,
- determine types of research appropriate for the intramural agencies to fund (some research priorities will not be funded by extramural programs),
- plan the content of future dietary surveys with an eye toward the future needs for the DRIs, and
- develop the food composition analytical methods and data that are essential in establishing DRI values.

Incentives or disincentives for private sector research merit some consideration. Clearly, food companies have provided valuable food composition data. Working relationships have been especially good when a particular company or group of companies has had a special interest in a nutrient. Thus, there can be very good incentives for developing more food composition data and including the private sector in that effort.

Legislation has led to some disincentives, especially as related to dietary supplements. Perhaps, with a different set of incentives, there might be more reason for pharmaceutical companies to invest in answering some of the fundamental nutrition research questions.

As a follow-up to points raised during the workshop, consideration might be given to incentives for developing software both for professional use and for educational purposes and to incentives for formula companies to address some of the questions raised that pertain to requirements of infants.

Responsibility for Leading the Research Agenda

In moving forward, who has responsibility for leading this research agenda? Dr. Woteki stated that, without question, the government agencies do; and the coordinating body that involves research and action agencies in both Canada and the United States holds promise. The Food and Nutrition Board continues to have important roles in the development of the type of research synthesis that has led to the DRIs, as a body for strategic planning in the areas of food and nutrition, and in convening groups that can move the questions forward. Nonetheless, Dr. Woteki takes the position that the major responsibility for implementation of the agenda rests with the funding agencies.

From her current perspective with a major food company, Dr. Woteki reemphasized the importance of the DRIs for public health and for policy applications, and she reemphasized how extremely important it is that the research base be defensible. Quoting Dr. Lindsay Allen, "This is serious stuff, and it deserves investment."

COMMENTS BY DENNIS M. BIER

This presentation addressed research opportunities, highlighting those related to new techniques. In addition, it briefly covered biomarkers for foods, ethical issues, and a systematic approach for setting ULs. In his opening remarks, Dr. Bier spoke about the logo of the Children's Nutrition Research Center at Baylor College of Medicine. That logo shows happy children eating. The joys of food provide a reason to solve some of the research questions raised—to allow people to enjoy what they eat.

Opportunities

To move the research forward, there is a need to communicate the excitement. For example, what is the real relevance of finding the answers to the questions? How can the research questions be framed in a way that gets agencies and researchers interested in them?

One approach would be to use the new tools (genomics, epigenomics, proteomics, and metabolomics) to capture the excitement in the questions and bring young people into the field. There is an urgency to determine the relevance to human health of some of the epigenetic regulation issues with dietary intake. At the time the recommendation was made to fortify grains with folic acid, for example, the epigenetic effects of methyl donors were unknown and did not enter the discussion at all.

Another approach to generate interest is to build on the experience of the clinical pharmacology specialty and to develop a new specialty called clinical nutricology. For example, clinical pharmacologists showed that (1) pharmacokinetics had relevance to direct human health and behavior in the use of drugs, (2) genotypes altered the metabolism of drugs in a way that was relevant to human beings, and (3) the interaction among drugs was important to their effects in human beings—in fact, components of diet such as grapefruit juice were important to the metabolism of drugs. The parallel content of clinical nutricology can be seen simply by changing the word *drug* to *nutrient* in the example above.

Biomarkers for Foods

Although the workshop gave much attention to the need for biomarkers and status indicators, Dr. Bier emphasized that there is also a need for biomarkers in foods. Food biomarkers could make it possible to know, for example, whether someone ate broccoli or not. Developing biomarkers in food could lead to a better independent assessment of dietary intake.

Ethical Issues

Participants raised a number of ethical issues during the workshop. Addressing them is extremely important to make it possible to conduct experiments related to the nutritional needs of children. For children, Dr.

Bier views the issue of safe study design to be of greater importance than developing the justification for the research. For studies relating to the ULs, developing the justification appears to be more important than the study design. Citing a specific example related to research relevant to ULs for amino acids, Dr. Bier indicated that, despite being given specific instructions on information needs for a symposium on amino acid science, only a small proportion of the invited scientists provided information on why they need to do specific studies.

Systematic Approach to a Decision Tree for Setting ULs

As his final comment, Dr. Bier stated that a systematic approach to a decision tree for setting ULs, as proposed by Dr. Sanford Miller, would be very helpful in improving the process for setting ULs.

DISCUSSION

No formal discussion occurred at the end of the session. However, earlier in the workshop, discussants raised points pertinent to the appropriateness of the DRI paradigm and methods for obtaining answers to research questions. These points are summarized below. These comments are not to be interpreted as consensus comments or recommendations.

The General Model

- The model suggests a level of precision that we are unlikely to have.
- The model is only as good as the indicators being measured. EARs were based on indicators having acceptable data, not on optimum nutrition. The model poses problems when an aim is chronic disease prevention.
- A new DRI committee may be helpful to address methods for setting DRIs for infants and children.
- The paradigm needs to be enlarged to include adaptations for DRIs for people who are ill. The DRIs are useful as long as illness does not change the requirement, but there has not been a

systematic examination of conditions for which changes in DRIs would be advisable. Considerable work has been done in medicine to determine the effects of specific conditions on nutrient requirements.

- The appropriateness of the model was questioned for food components that have not yet been addressed (e.g., phytochemicals).

Method Used for Setting the RDA

Several discussants pointed out that variability in requirements is assumed rather than known for most nutrients. Setting the RDA at four rather than two standard deviations above the EAR, as suggested by Dr. Hathcock, would cover a higher percentage of the population and might make sense from the viewpoint of not missing 2 to 3 percent of the population. In some cases, however, a higher RDA could make it unrealistic to achieve the RDA using traditional foods. The people who are most likely to take multivitamin-mineral supplements are the people with the highest nutrient intakes, leading to intakes that might be high enough to be of concern (see third bullet in this set).

Considerable discussion centered on approaches to cover a substantial proportion of the population with a polymorphism: (1) increase the RDA or (2) recommend genetic testing and individualize the requirement? Dr. Stover clarified that individualization of requirements based on results from genetic testing probably would not be necessary as long as there is enough room between the RDA and the UL. In setting the RDA, one would include consideration of the genetic variance, similar to what was done in setting the vitamin B_{12} RDA for persons age 50 years and older. In theory, there is no need to individualize requirements unless one person's requirement is another person's UL. Dr. Rosenberg commented that bimodal distributions associated with the presence of polymorphisms, if not embedded in the population, might result in a need to change the model. He believes however, that the variability may be embedded in the variability of the population.

Dr. Zeisel believes that the measurement of single nucleotide polymorphism (SNPs) will be relatively inexpensive (perhaps $100 to obtain 50,000 SNPs) and widely available within 5 years. Information about SNPs is valid over one's lifetime. Thus, the practice of nutrition may well involve telling individuals that they have certain SNPs that increase their requirements. Dr. Zeisel would like the DRI process to consider setting the RDA at a level that covers essentially everyone but also noting that the RDA would be lower for people without the SNPs. Several discussants expressed concern about possible side effects from recommending too high an intake. For example, if the nutrient affects perinatal programming, there could be unforeseen adverse consequences of treating everyone with a large dose.

Communication Problems

Discussants mentioned a variety of ways in which the DRIs can lead to communication problems, such as the following:

- Lack of coverage of a large number of people in a country assuming that the RDA covers 97 to 98 percent of the population—the RDA may be viewed as too low
- Needs of a given individual may be much lower than the RDA—the RDA may be viewed as too high
- High percentages of the population who have intakes of selected nutrients that fall below the EAR—the EAR may be viewed as too high
- Different meanings of the AI
- Lack of correspondence between the carbohydrate RDA and AMDR

Finding Answers to Questions

Dr. Joanne Guthrie of the Economic Research Service (ERS) of the USDA commented that resources are available for testing some of the methods proposed in the DRI Assessment Report (IOM, 2000a) and the DRI Planning Report (IOM, 2003a). Relevant databases are available. The Food Assistance and Nutrition Research Program of the ERS and grants programs in some other agencies support research of this type. Dr. Guthrie encouraged researchers to collaborate with new partners, such as biostatisticians, to make use of the databases. Understanding distributions by analyzing existing data, for example, would be a good first step.

References

Abrams SA, Griffin IJ, Hawthorne KM, Chen Z, Gunn SK, Wilde M, Darlington G, Shypailo RJ, Ellis KJ. 2005. Vitamin D receptor Fok1 polymorphisms affect calcium absorption, kinetics, and bone mineralization rates during puberty. *J Bone Miner Res* 20(6): 945–953.

Age-Related Eye Disease Study Research Group. 2001. A randomized, placebo-controlled, clinical trial of high-dose supplementation with vitamins C and E, beta carotene, and zinc for age-related macular degeneration and vision loss: AREDS report no. 8. *Arch Ophthalmol* 119(10):1417–1436.

Ajani UA, Ford ES, Mokdad AH. 2004. Dietary fiber and C-reactive protein: findings from National Health and Nutrition Examination Survey data. *J Nutr* 134(5):1181–1185.

Armas, LAG, Hollis BW, Hearney, RP. 2004. Vitamin D2 is much less effective than vitamin D3 in humans. *J Clin Endocrinol Metab* 89:5387–5391.

Ascherio A, Rimm EB, Hernan MA, Giovannucci EL, Kawachi I, Stampfer MJ, Willett WC. 1998. Intake of potassium, magnesium, calcium, and fiber, and risk of stroke among US men. *Circulation* 98(12):1198–1204.

Ashfield-Watt PA, Pullin CH, Whiting JM, Clark ZE, Moat SJ, Newcombe RG, Burr ML, Lewis MJ, Powers HJ, McDowell IF. 2002. Methylenetratrahydrofolate reductase 677C→T genotype modulates homocysteine responses to a folate-rich diet or a low-dose folic acid supplement: a randomized controlled trial. *Am J Clin Nutr* 76(1):180–186.

Barbagallo M, Gupta RK, Dominguez LJ, Resnick LM. 2000. Cellular ionic alterations with age: Relation to hypertension and diabetes. *J Am Geriatr Soc* 48(9):1111–1116.

Baron JA, Cole BF, Mott L, Haile R, Grau M, Church TR, Beck GJ, Greenberg ER. 2003. Neoplastic and antineoplastic effects of beta-carotene on colorectal adenoma recurrence: Results of a randomized trial. *J Natl Cancer Inst* 95(10):717–722.

Basiotis PP, Welsh SO, Cronin FJ, Kelsay JL, Mertz W. 1987. Number of days of food intake records required to estimate individual and group nutrient intakes with defined confidence. *J Nutr* 117:1638–1641.

Beaton GH. 1994. Criteria of an adequate diet. In: Shils ME, Olson JA, Shike M, eds. *Modern Nutrition in Health and Disease*, 8th edition. Philadelphia: Lea & Febiger. 1491–1505.

Beltran-Aguilar ED, Barker LK, Canto MT, Dye BA, Gooch BF, Griffin SO, Hyman J, Jaramillo F, Kingman A, Nowjack-Raymer R, Selwitz RH, Wu T. 2005. Centers for Disease Control and Prevention (CDC). Surveillance for dental caries, dental sealants, tooth retention, edentulism, and enamel fluorosis: United States, 1988–1994 and 1999–2002. *MMWR Surveill Summ* 54(3):1–43.

Benyo Z, Gille A, Kero J, Csiky M, Suchankova MC, Nusing RM, Moers A, Pfeffer K, Offermanns S. 2005. GPR109A (PUMA-G/HM74A) mediates nicotinic acid-induced flushing. *J Clin Invest* 115(12):3634–3640.

Berkey CS, Rockett HR, Field AE, Gillman MW, Colditz GA. 2004. Sugar-added beverages and adolescent weight change. *Obes Res* 12:778–788.

Borghi L, Schianchi T, Meschi T, Guerra A, Allegri F, Maggiore U, Novarini A. 2002. Comparison of two diets for the prevention of recurrent stones in idiopathic hypercalciuria. *N Engl J Med* 346(2):77–84.

Brindle JT, Antti H, Holmes E, Tranter G, Nicholson JK, Bethell HW, Clarke S, Schofield PM, McKilligin E, Mosedale DE, Grainger DJ. 2002. Rapid and noninvasive diagnosis of the presence and severity of coronary heart disease using 1H-NMR-based metabonomics. *Nat Med* 8:1439–1445. Erratum in: Nat Med 2003 Apr:9(4):477.

Chan JM, Stampfer MJ, Ma J, Rimm EB, Willett WC, Giovannucci EL. 1999. Supplemental vitamin E intake and prostate cancer risk in a large cohort of men in the United States. *Cancer Epidemiol Biomarkers Prev* 8(10):893–899.

Chapuy MC, Arlot ME, Duboeuf F, Brun J, Crouzet B, Arnaud S, Delmas PD, Meunier PJ. 1992. Vitamin D3 and calcium to prevent hip fractures in elderly women. *N Engl J Med* 327(23):1637–1642.

Chapuy MC, Pamphile R, Paris E, Kempf C, Schlichting M, Arnaud S, Garnero P, Meunier PJ. 2002. Combined calcium and vitamin D3 supplementation in elderly women: Confirmation of reversal of secondary hyperparathyroidism and hip fracture risk: The Decalyos II study. *Osteoporos Int* 13(3):257–264.

Chen J, Zhao X, Zhang X, Yin S, Piao J, Huo J, Yu B, Qu N, Lu Q, Wang S, Chen C. 2005. Studies on the effectiveness of NaFeEDTA-fortified soy sauce in controlling iron deficiency: A population-based intervention trial. *Food Nutr Bulletin* 26:177–189.

Chiang EP, Selhub J, Bagley PJ, Dallal G, Roubenoff R. 2005a. Pyridoxine supplementation corrects vitamin B6 deficiency but does not improve inflammation in patients with rheumatoid arthritis. *Arthritis Res Ther* 7(6):R1404–R1411.

Chiang EP, Smith DE, Selhub J, Dallal G, Wang YC, Roubenoff R. 2005b. Inflammation causes tissue-specific depletion of vitamin B6. *Arthritis Res Ther* 7(6):R1254–R1262.

Cho E, Zeisel SH, Jacques P, Selhub J, Dougherty L, Colditz GA, Willett WC. 2006. Dietary choline and betaine assessed by food-frequency questionnaire in relation to plasma total homocysteine concentration in the Framingham Offspring Study. *Am J Clin Nutr* 83:905-911.

Clark LC, Combs GF Jr, Turnbull BW, Slate EH, Chalker DK, Chow J, Davis LS, Glover RA, Graham GF, Gross EG, Krongrad A, Lesher JL Jr, Park HK, Sanders BB Jr, Smith CL, Taylor JR. 1996. Effects of selenium supplementation for cancer prevention in patients with carcinoma of the skin. A randomized controlled trial. Nutritional Prevention of Cancer Study Group. *JAMA* 276(24):1957–1963. Erratum in: *JAMA.* 1997, 277(19):1520.

Cockayne S, Adamson J, Lanham-New S, Shearer MJ, Gilbody S, Torgerson DJ. 2006. Vitamin K and the prevention of fractures: Systematic review and meta-analysis of randomized controlled trials. *Arch Intern Med* 166(12):1256–1261.

COMA (Committee on Medical Aspects of Food Policy). 1991. *Dietary Reference Values for Food Energy and Nutrients for the United Kingdom.* Report on Health and Social Subjects, No. 41. London: Her Majesty's Stationery Office.

Cook JD, Flowers CH, Skikne BS. 2003. The quantitative assessment of body iron. *Blood* 101:3359–3363.

Cooney CA, Dave AA, Wolff GL. 2002. Maternal methyl supplements in mice affect epigenetic variation and DNA methylation of offspring. *J Nutr* 132:2392S–2400S.

Corella D, Qi L, Soreli JV, Godoy D, Portoles O, Coltell O, Greenberg AS, Ordovas JM. 2005. Obese subjects carrying the 11482G>A polymorphism at the perilipin locus are resistant to weight loss after dietary energy restriction. *J Clin Endocrinol Metab* 90(9):5121–5126.

Cosmetic Ingredient Review Expert Panel. 2005. Final report of the safety assessment of niacinamide and niacin. *Int J Toxicol* 24(suppl 5):1–31.

Cummings JH. 1993. The effect of dietary fiber on fecal weight and composition. In: Spiller GA, ed. *CRC Handbook of Dietary Fiber in Human Nutrition*, 2nd ed. Boca Raton, FL: CRC Press.

Dawson-Hughes B, Harris SS, Krall EA, Dallal GE. 1997. Effect of calcium and vitamin D supplementation on bone density in men and women 65 years of age or older. *N Engl J Med* 337(10):670–676.

da Costa KA, Kozyreva OG, Song J, Galanko JA, Fischer LM, Zeisel SH. 2006a. Common genetic polymorphisms affect the human requirement for the nutrient choline. *FASEB J* 20:1336–1344.

da Costa KA, Niculescu MD, Craciunescu CN, Fischer LM, Zeisel SH. 2006b. Choline deficiency increases lymphocyte apoptosis and DNA damage in humans. *Am J Clin Nutr* 84(1):88–94.

de Romana DL, Lonnerdal B, Brown KH. 2003. Absorption of zinc from wheat products fortified with iron and either zinc sulfate or zinc oxide. *Am J Clin Nutr* 78:279–283.

Devaney B, Ziegler P, Pac S, Karwe V, Barr SI. 2004. Nutrient intakes of infants and toddlers. *J Am Diet Assoc* 104(1 Suppl 1):s14–21.

Devirian TA, Volpe SL. 2003. The physiological effects of dietary boron. *Crit Rev Food Sci Nutr* 43:219–231.

DHHS/USDA (Department of Health and Human Services/U.S. Department of Agriculture). 2004. *Report of the Dietary Guidelines Advisory Committee on the Dietary Guidelines for Americans, 2005 to the Secretary of Health and Human Services and the Secretary of Agriculture.* [Online]. Available: http://www.healthierus.gov/dietary guidelines [accessed September 15, 2006].

DHHS/USDA. 2005. *Dietary Guidelines for Americans 2005*. 6th ed. Washington, DC: U.S. Government Printing Office. GPO No 001-000-04719-1.

Dolinoy DC, Weidman JR, Waterland RA, Jirtle RL. 2006. Maternal genistein alters coat color and protects Avy mouse offspring from obesity by modifying the fetal epigenome. *Environ Health Perspect* 114(4):567–572.

Domellof M, Lonnerdal B, Abrams SA, Hernell O. 2002. Iron absorption in breast-fed infants: Effects of age, iron status, iron supplements, and complementary foods. *Am J Clin Nutr* 76(1):198–204.

Domellof M, Lonnerdal B, Dewey KG, Cohen RJ, Hernell O. 2004 Iron, zinc, and copper concentrations in breast milk are independent of maternal mineral status. *Am J Clin Nutr* 79(1):111–5. Erratum in: *Am J Clin Nutr* 2004 80(6):1669.

Duffield-Lillico AJ, Reid ME, Turnbull BW, Combs GF Jr, Slate EH, Fischbach LA, Marshall JR, Clark LC. 2002. Baseline characteristics and the effect of selenium supplementation on cancer incidence in a randomized clinical trial: A summary report of the Nutritional Prevention of Cancer Trial. *Cancer Epidemiol Biomarkers Prev* 11(7):630–639.

FAO/WHO/UNU (Food and Agriculture Organization of the United Nations/World Health Organization/United Nations Association). 1985. *Energy and Protein Requirements. Report of a Joint FAO/WHO/UNA Expert Consultation*. Technical Report Series. No. 724. Geneva, Switzerland: WHO.

FAO/WHO (Food and Agriculture Organization and World Health Organization), The International Programme on Chemical Safety. 2005. *A Model for Establishing Upper Levels of Intake for Nutrients and Related Substances: Report of a Joint FAO/WHO Technical Workshop on Nutrient Risk Assessment*.[Online]. Available: http://www.who.int/ipcs/methods/nra/en/index.html [accessed September 15, 2006].

Feskanich D, Singh V, Willett WC, Colditz GA. 2002. Vitamin A intake and hip fractures among postmenopausal women. *JAMA* 287(1): 47–54.

Fine KD, Schiller LR. 1999. GAG technical review on the evaluation and management of chronic diarrhea. *Gastroenterology* 116:1464–1486.

Garza C, Scrimshaw NS, Young VR. 1977. Human protein requirements: A long-term metabolic nitrogen balance study in young men to evaluate the 1973 FAO/WHO safe level of egg protein intake. *Br J Nutr* 37(3):403–420.

Giovannucci E, Liu Y, Rimm EB, Hollis BW, Fuchs CS, Stampfer MJ, Willett WC. 2006. Prospective study of predictors of vitamin D status and cancer incidence and mortality in men. *J Natl Cancer Inst* 98:451–459.

Gori AM, Sofi F, Corsi AM, Gazzini A, Sestini I, Lauretani F, Bandinelli S, Gensini GF, Ferrucci L, Abbate R. 2006. Predictors of vitamin B6 and folate concentrations in older persons: The InCHIANTI study. *Clin Chem* 52(7):1318–1324.

Goulding A, Cannan R, Williams SM, Gold EJ, Taylor RW, Lewis-Barned NJ. 1998. Bone mineral density in girls with forearm fractures. *J Bone Miner Res* 13:143–148.

Grant AM, Avenell A, Campbell MK, McDonald AM, MacLennan GS, McPherson GC, Anderson FH, Cooper C, Francis RM, Donaldson C, Gillespie WJ, Robinson CM, Torgerson DJ, Wallace WA, RECORD Trial Group. 2005. Oral vitamin D3 and calcium for secondary prevention of low-trauma fractures in elderly people (Randomised Evaluation of Calcium Or vitamin D—RECORD): A randomised placebo-controlled trial. *Lancet* 365(9471):1621–1680.

Guenther BD, Sheppard CA, Tran P, Rozen R, Matthews RG, Ludwig ML. 1999. The structure and properties of methylenetetrahydrofolate reductase from *Escherichia coli* suggest how folate ameliorates human hyperhomocysetinemoa. *Nat Struct Biol* 6(4):359–365.

Guinotte CL, Burns MG, Axume JA, Hata H, Urrutia TF, Alamilla A, McCabe D, Singgih A, Cogger EA, Caudill MA. 2003. Methylenetetrahydrofolate reductate 667C→T variant modulates folate status response to controlled folate intakes in young women. *J Nutr* 133:1272–1280.

Haddad JG, Chyu K. 1971. Competitive protein-binding radioassay for 25 hydroxychol-calciferol. *J Clin Endocrinol Metab* 33:992–995.

Hadley KB, Johnson LK, Hunt JR. 2006. Absorption by healthy women is not associated with either serum or urinary prohepcidin. *Am J Clin Nutr* 84:150–155.

Hambidge KM, Krebs NF, Westcott JE, Miller LV. 2006. Changes in zinc absorption during development. *J Pediatr* 149(suppl 3):64–68.

Haskell MJ, Jamil KM, Hassan F, Peerson JM, Hossain MI, Fuchs GJ, Brown KH. 2004. Daily consumption of Indian spinach (*Basella alba*) or sweet potatoes has a positive effect on total-body vitamin A stores in Bangladeshi men. *Am J Clin Nutr* 80(3):705–714.

He FJ, Markandu ND, Coltart R, Barron J, MacGregor GA. 2005. Effect of short-term supplementation of potassium chloride and potassium citrate on blood pressure in hypertensives. *Hypertension* 45(4):571–574.

Heaney, RP, Davies KM, Chen TC, Holick MF, Barger-Lux MJ. 2003. Human serum 25–hydroxycholecalciferol response to extended oral dosing with cholecalciferol. *Am J Clin Nutr* 77:204–210.

Health Canada (Health Canada, Health Products and Food Branch, Office of Nutrition Policy and Promotion). 2006. *Canadian Community Health Survey Cycle 2.2, Nutrition (2004): A Guide to Accessing and Interpreting the Data.* Ottawa, Ontario: Health Canada. [Online]. Available: http://www.hc-sc.gc.ca/fn-an/surveill/nutrition/commun/index_e.html (accessed August 20, 2006).

Herman S, Griffin IJ, Suwarti S, Ernawati F, Permaesih D, Pambudi D, Abrams SA. 2002. Cofortification of iron-fortified flour with zinc sulfate, but not zinc oxide, decreases iron absorption in Indonesian children. *Am J Clin Nutr* 76:813–817.

Hollis, BW, Wagner CL. 2004. Vitamin D requirements during lactation: High-dose maternal supplementation as therapy to prevent hypovitaminosis D for both the mother and the nursing infant. *Am J Clin Nutr* 80:1752S–1758S.

Hoppe M, Hulthen L, Hallberg L. 2003. Serum iron concentration as a tool to measure relative iron absorption from elemental iron powders in man. *Scand J Clin Lab Invest* 63:489–496.

Hurrell R, Bothwell T, Cook JD, Dary O, Davidsson L, Fairweather-Tait S, Hallberg L, Lynch S, Rosado J, Walter T, Whittaker P. 2002. The usefulness of elemental iron for cereal flour fortification: A SUSTAIN Task Force report. Sharing United States Technology to Aid in the Improvement of Nutrition. *Nutr Rev* 60:391–406.

Hustad S, Ueland PM, Vollset SE, Zhang Y, Bjorke-Monsen AL, Schneede J. 2000. Riboflavin as a determinant of plasma total homocysteine: Effect of modification by the methylenetetrahydrofolate reductase C677T polymorphism. *Clin Chem* 46(8 Pt 1):1065–1071.

International Zinc Nutrition Consultative Group. 2004. Assessment of the risk of zinc deficiency in populations and options for its control. *Food and Nutrition Bulletin* 25 (1, Supp 2):S99–S129.

IOM (Institute of Medicine). 1994. *How Should the Recommended Dietary Allowances Be Revised?* Washington, DC: National Academy Press.

IOM. 1997. *Dietary Reference Intakes for Calcium, Phosphorus, Magnesium, Vitamin D, and Fluoride.* Washington, DC: National Academy Press.

IOM. 1998a. *Dietary Reference Intakes for Thiamin, Riboflavin, Niacin, Vitamin B6, Folate, Vitamin B12, Pantothenic Acid, Biotin, and Choline*. Washington, DC: National Academy Press.

IOM 1998b. *A Risk Assessment Model for Establishing Upper Intake Levels for Nutrients*. Washington, DC: National Academy Press.

IOM. 2000a. *Dietary Reference Intakes: Applications in Dietary Assessment*. Washington, DC: National Academy Press.

IOM. 2000b. *Dietary Reference Intakes for Vitamin C, Vitamin E, Selenium, and Carotenoids.* Washington, DC: National Academy Press.

IOM. 2001. *Dietary Reference Intakes for Vitamin A, Vitamin K, Arsenic, Boron, Chromium, Copper, Iodine, Iron, Manganese, Molybdenum, Nickel, Silicon, Vanadium, and Zinc.* Washington, DC: National Academies Press.

IOM. 2002/2005. *Dietary Reference Intakes for Energy, Carbohydrate, Fiber, Fat, Fatty Acids, Cholesterol, Protein, and Amino Acids.* Washington, DC: National Academies Press.

IOM. 2003a. *Dietary Reference Intakes: Applications in Dietary Planning.* Washington, DC: National Academies Press.

IOM. 2003b. *Dietary Reference Intakes: Guiding Principles for Nutrition Labeling and Fortification.* Washington, DC: National Academies Press.

IOM. 2005. *Dietary Reference Intakes for Water, Potassium, Sodium, Chloride, and Sulfate.* Washington, DC: National Academies Press.

IOM. 2006a. *Dietary Reference Intakes: The Essential Guide to Nutrient Requirements*. Washington, DC: National Academies Press.

IOM. 2006b. *Mineral Requirements for Military Personnel; Levels Needed for Cognitive and Physical Performance During Garrison Training*. Washington, DC: National Academies Press.

IOM. 2006c. *WIC Food Packages: Time for a Change*. Washington, DC: National Academies Press.

Jackson RD, LaCroix AZ, Gass M, Wallace RB, Robbins J, Lewis CE, Bassford T, Beresford SA, Black HR, Blanchette P, Bonds DE, Brunner RL, Brzyski RG, Caan B, Cauley JA, Chlebowski RT, Cummings SR, Granek I, Hays J, Heiss G, Hendrix SL, Howard BV, Hsia J, Hubbell FA, Johnson KC, Judd H, Kotchen JM, Kuller LH, Langer RD, Lasser NL, Limacher MC, Ludlam S, Manson JE, Margolis KL, McGowan J, Ockene JK, O'Sullivan MJ, Phillips L, Prentice RL, Sarto GE, Stefanick ML, Van Horn L, Wactawski-Wende J, Whitlock E, Anderson GL, Assaf AR, Barad D; Women's

Health Initiative Investigators. 2006. Calcium plus vitamin D supplementation and the risk of fractures. *N Engl J Med* 354(7):669–83. Erratum in: *N Engl J Med* 2006 354(10):1102.

Jacques PF, Taylor A, Moeller S, Hankinson SE, Rogers G, Tung W, Ludovico J, Willet WC, Chylack LT Jr. 2005. Long-term nutrient intake and 5-year change in nuclear lens opacities. *Arch Ophthalmol* 123(4):517–526.

Jalla S, Westcott J, Steirn M, Miller LV, Bell M, Krebs NF. 2002. Zinc absorption and exchangeable zinc pool sizes in breast-fed infants fed meat or cereal as first complementary food. *J Pediatr Gastr Nutr* 34:35–41.

Kang SS, Zhou J, Wong PW, Kowalisyn J, Strokosch G. 1988. Intermediate homocysteinemia: a thermolabile variant of methylene-tetrahydrofolate reductase. *Am J Hum Genet* 43(4):414–421.

Kelly P, McPartlin J, Goggins M, Weir DG, Scott JM. 1997. Unmetabolized folic acid in serum: Acute studies in subjects consuming fortified food and supplements. *Am J Clin Nutr* 65(6):1790–1795.

Kirsh VA, Hayes RB, Mayne ST, Chatterjee N, Subar AF, Dixon LB, Albanes D, Andriole GL, Urban DA, Peters U; PLCO Trial. 2006. Supplemental and dietary vitamin E, beta-carotene, and vitamin C intakes and prostate cancer risk. *J Natl Cancer Inst* 98(4):245–254.

Kohlmeier M, da Costa KA, Fischer LM, Zeisel SH. 2005. Genetic variation of folate-mediated one-carbon transfer pathway predicts susceptibility to choline deficiency in humans. *Proc Natl Acad Sci USA* 102:16025-16030.

Krebs NF, Westcott JE. 2002. Zinc and breast-fed infants: If and when is there a risk of deficiency? In: Davis MK, Isaacs CE, Hanson LA, Wright AL, eds. *Integrating Population Outcomes, Biological Mechanisms and Research Methods in the Study of Human Milk and Lactation*. New York: Kluwer Academic/Plenum Publishers.

Krebs NF, Westcott JE, Butler N, Robinson C, Bell M, Hambidge KM. 2006. Meat as a first complementary food for breast-fed infants: Feasibility and impact on zinc intake and status. *J Pediatr Gastroenter Nutr* 42:207–214.

Lahoz C, Schaefer EJ, Cupples LA, Wilson PW, Levy D, Osgood D, Parpos S, Pedro-Botet J, Daly JA, Ordovas JM. 2001. Apolipoprotein E genotype and cardiovascular disease in the Framingham Heart Study. *Atherosclerosis* 154(3):529–537.

Lembo A, Camilleri M. 2003. Chronic constipation. *N Engl J Med* 349:1360–1368.

Lips P Graafmans WC, Ooms ME, Bezemer PD, Bouter LM. 1996. Vitamin D supplementation and fracture incidence in elderly persons. A randomized, placebo-controlled clinical trial. *Ann Intern Med* 124:400–406.

Liu, PT, Stenger S, Li H, Wenzel L, Tan BH, Krutzik S, Ochoa MT, Schauber J, Wu K, Meinken C, Kamen DL, Wagner M, Bals R, Steinmeyer A, Zugel U, Modlin RL. 2006. Toll-like receptor triggering of a vitamin D-mediated human antimicrobial response. *Science* 311:1770–1773.

Liuzzi JP, Cousins RJ. 2004. Mammalian zinc transporters. *Annu Rev Nutr* 24:151–172.

Lopez de Romana D, Salazar M, Hambidge KM, Penny ME, Peerson JM, Krebs NF, Brown KH. 2005. Longitudinal measurements of zinc absorption in Peruvian children consuming wheat products fortified with iron only or iron and 1 of 2 amounts of zinc. *Am J Clin Nutr* 81:637–647.

Lopez-Ridaura R, Willett WC, Rimm EB, Liu S, Stampfer MJ, Manson JE. 2004. Magnesium intake and risk of type 2 diabetes in men and women. *Diabetes Care* 27(1):134–140.

Luft FC, Rankin LI, Bloch R, Weyman AE, Willis LR, Murray RH, Grim CE, Weinberger MH. 1979. Cardiovascular and humoral responses to extremes of sodium intake in normal black and white men. *Circulation* 60:697–706.

Ma Y, Griffith JA, Chasan-Taber L, Olendzki BC, Jackson E, Stanek EJ 3rd, Li W, Pagoto SL, Hafner AR, Ockene IS. 2006. Association between dietary fiber and serum C-reactive protein. *Am J Clin Nutr* 83(4):760–766.

Matkovic V, Goel PK, Badenhop-Stevens NE, Landoll JD, Li B, Ilich JZ, Skugor M, Nagode LA, Mobley SL, Ha EJ, Hangartner TN, Clairmont A. 2005. Calcium supplementation and bone mineral density in females from childhood to young adulthood: A randomized controlled trial. *Am J Clin Nutr* 81:175–188.

Melse-Boonstra A, Holm PI, Ueland PM, Olthof M, Clarke R, Verhoef P. 2005. Betaine concentration as a determinant of fasting total homocysteine concentrations and the effect of folic acid supplementation on betaine concentrations. *Am J Clin Nutr* 81:1378-1382.

Meyer HE, Smedshaug GB, Kvaavik E, Falch JA, Tverdal A, Pedersen JI. 2002. Can vitamin D supplementation reduce the risk of fracture in the elderly? A randomized controlled trial. *J Bone Miner Res* 17(4):709–715.

Miller EG III, Pastor-Barriuso R, Dalal D, Riemersma RA, Appel LJ, Guallar E. 2005. Meta-analysis: High-dosage vitamin E supplementation may increase all-cause mortality. *Ann Intern Med* 142: 37-46.

Morgan HD, Sutherland, HG, Martin DI, Whitelaw E. 1999. Epigenetic inheritance at the agouti locus in the mouse. *Nat Genet* 23(3): 314–318.

Morris RC Jr, Sebastian A, Forman A, Tanaka M, Schmidlin O. 1999. Normotensive salt-sensitivity: Effects of race and dietary potassium. *Hypertension* 33:18–23.

Moshfegh A, Goldman J, Cleveland L. 2005 *What We Eat in America, NHANES 2001–2002: Usual Nutrient Intakes from Food Compared to Dietary Reference Intakes*. U.S. Department of Agriculture, Agricultural Research Service. [Online]. Available: http://www.ars.usda.gov/SP2UserFiles/Place/12355000/pdf/usualintaketables2001-02.pdf (accessed September 10, 2006).

Mrdjenovic G, Levitsky DA. 2003. Nutritional and energetic consequences of sweetened drink consumption in 6- to 13-year-old children. *J Pediatr* 142:604–610.

Narang MA, Dumas R, Ayer LM, Gravel RA. 2004. Reduced histone biotinylation in multiple carboxylase deficiency patients: A nuclear role for holocarboxylase synthetase. *Human Molecular Genet* 13: 15–23.

Nemeth E, Ganz T. 2006. Regulation of iron metabolism by hepcidin. *Annu Rev Nutr* 26:323–342.

NRC (National Research Council). 1943. *Recommended Dietary Allowances. Report of the Food and Nutrition Board.* Reprint and Circular Series No. 115. Washington, DC: National Research Council.

NRC. 1989a. *Diet and Health.* Washington, DC: National Academy Press.

NRC. 1989b. *Recommended Dietary Allowances.* Washington, DC: National Academy Press.

O'Brien MM, Kiely M, Harrington KE, Robson PJ, Strain JJ, Flynn A. 2001. The North/South Ireland Food Consumption Survey: Vitamin intakes in 18- to 64-year-old adults. *Public Health Nutr* 4(5A):1069–1079.

Oettle GJ. 1991. Effect of moderate exercise on bowel habit. *Gut* 32(8):941–944.

Phillips SM, Bandini LG, Naumova EN, Cyr H, Colclough S, Dietz WH, Must A. 2004. Energy-dense snack food intake in adolescence: Longitudinal relationship to weight and fatness. *Obesity Res* 12: 461–472.

Prince RL, Devine A, Dhaliwal SS, Dick IM. 2006. Effects of calcium supplementation on clinical fracture and bone structure: Results of a 5-year, double-blind, placebo-controlled trial in elderly women. *Arch Intern Med* 166(8):869–875.

Rehman, P. 1994. Subclinical rickets and recurrent infection. *J Tropical Pediatr* 40:58.

Ribaya-Mercado JD, Solon FS, Solon MA, Cabal-Barza MA, Perfecto CS, Tang G, Solon JA, Fjeld CR, Russell RM. 2000. Bioconversion of plant steroids to vitamin A in Filipino school-aged children varies inversely with vitamin A status. *Am J Clin Nutr* 72(2):455–465.

Rocchietta, S. 1960. Notes for a history of physiotherapy. Niel Ryberg Finsen (1860–1904), pioneer of modern phototherapy. *Minerva Med* 51:966–968.

Rude RK, Gruber HE, Norton HJ, Wei LY, Frausto A, Mills BG. 2004. Bone loss induced by dietary magnesium reduction to 10% of the nutrient requirement in rats is associated with increased release of substance P and tumor necrosis factor-alpha. *J Nutr* 134(1):79–85.

Rude RK, Gruber HE, Norton HJ, Wei LY, Frausto A, Kilburn J. 2005. Dietary magnesium reduction to 25% of nutrient requirement disrupts bone and mineral metabolism in the rat. *Bone* 37(2): 211–219.

Rude RK, Gruber HE, Norton HJ, Wei LY, Frausto A, Kilburn J. 2006. Reduction of dietary magnesium by only 50% in the rat disrupts bone and mineral metabolism. *Osteoporos Int* 17(7):1022–1032.

Shaw GM, Carmichael SL, Yang W, Selvin S, Schaffer DM. 2004. Periconceptional dietary intake of choline and betaine and neural tube defects in offspring. *Am J Epidemiol* 160(2):102–109.

Shaw GM, Carmichael SL, Laurent C, Rasmussen SA. 2006. Maternal nutrient intakes and risk of orofacial clefts. *Epidemiology* 17(3): 285–291.

Sowers M, Whitford GM, Clark MK, Jannausch ML. 2005. Elevated serum fluoride concentrations in women are not related to fractures and bone mineral density. *J Nutr* 135(9):2247–2252.

Stanley JS, Griffin JB, Zempleni J. 2001. Biotinylation of histones in human cells. Effects of cell proliferation. *Eur J Biochem* 268:5424–5429.

Steingrimsdottir L, Gunnarsson O, Indridason OS, Franzson L, Sigurdsson G. 2005. Relationship between serum parathyroid hormone levels, vitamin D sufficiency, and calcium intake. *JAMA* 294(18):2336–2341.

Suitor CW, Gleason PM. 2002. Using Dietary Reference Intake-based methods to estimate the prevalence of inadequate nutrient intake school-aged children. *J Am Diet Assoc* 102(4):530–536.

Swain JH, Newman SM, Hunt JR. 2003. Bioavailability of elemental iron powders to rats is less than bakery-grade ferrous sulfate and predicted by iron solubility and particle surface area. *J Nutr* 133:3546–3552.

Tang G, Gu X, Hu S, Xu Q, Qin J, Doinikowski GG, Feld CR, Gao X, Russell RM, Yin S. 1999. Green and yellow vegetables can maintain body stores of vitamin A in Chinese children. *Am J Clin Nutr* 70(6):1069–1076.

Tang G, Qin J, Doinikowski GG, Russell RM, Grusak MA. 2005. Spinach or carrots can supply significant amounts of vitamin A as assessed by feeding with intrinsically deuterated vegetables. *Am J Clin Nutr* 82(4):821–828.

Tooze JA, Subar AF, Thompson FE, Troiano R, Schatzkin A, Kipnis V. 2004. Psychosocial predictors of energy underreporting in a large doubly labeled water study. *Am J Clin Nutr* 79(5):795–804.

Trivedi DP, Doll R, Khaw KT. 2003. Effect of four monthly oral vitamin D3 (cholecalciferol) supplementation on fractures and mortality in men and women living in the community: Randomised double blind controlled trial. *BMJ* 326(7387):469.

Troen AM, Mitchell B, Sorensen B, Wener MH, Johnston A, Wood B, Selhub J, McTiernan A, Yasui Y, Oral E, Potter JD, Ulrich CM. 2006. Unmetabolized folic acid in plasma is associated with reduced natural killer cell cytotoxicity among postmenopausal women. *J Nutr* 136(1):189–194.

Tucker DM, Sandstead HH, Logan GM Jr, Klevay LM, Mahalko J, Johnson LK, Inman L, Inglett GE. 1981. Dietary fiber and personality factors as determinants of stool output. *Gastroenterology*. 81(5):879–883.

USDA (United States Department of Agriculture). 2005. MyPyramid: Steps to a Healthier You. [Online]. Available: http://www.mypyramid.gov. (accessed September 9, 2006).

Van Thuy P, Berger J, Nakanishi Y, Khan NC, Lynch S, Dixon P. 2005. The use of NaFeEDTA–fortified fish sauce is an effective tool for controlling iron deficiency in women of childbearing age in rural Vietnam. *J Nutr* 135:2596–2601.

Vieth R, Chan PC, MacFarlane GD. 2001. Efficacy and safety of vitamin D3 intake exceeding the lowest observed adverse effect level. *Am J Clin Nutr* 73(2):288–294.

Virtamo J, Pietinen P, Huttunen JK, Korhonen P, Malila N, Virtanen MJ, Albanes D, Taylor PR, Albert P; ATBC Study Group. 2003. Incidence of cancer and mortality following alpha-tocopherol and beta-carotene supplementation: a postintervention follow-up. *JAMA* 290(4):476–485.

Wagner CL, Hulsey TC, Fanning D, Ebeling M, Hollis BW. 2006. High dose vitamin D3 supplementation in a cohort of breastfeeding mothers and their infants: a six months follow-up pilot study. *J Breastfeeding Medicine* 33:992-995.

Waterland RA, Jirtle RL. 2003. Transposable elements: targets for early nutritional effects on epigenetic gene regulation. *Mol Cell Biol* 23(15):5293–5300.

Wise A, Foord SM, Fraser NJ, Barnes AA, Elshourbagy N, Eilert M, Ignar DM, Murdock PR, Steplewski K, Green A, Brown AJ, Dowell SJ, Szekeres PG, Hassall DG, Marshall FH, Wilson S, Pike NB. 2003. Molecular identification of high and low affinity receptors for nicotinic acid. *J Biol Chem* 278(11):9869–9874.

Younes-Mhenni S, Derex L, Berruyer M, Nighoghossian N, Philippeau F, Saltzmann M, Trouillas P. 2004. Large-artery stroke in a young patient with Crohn's disease. Rose of vitamin B6 deficiency-induced hyperhomocysteinemia. *J Neur Sci* (1–2): 113–115.

Zimmermann MB, Winichagoon P, Gowachirapant S, Hess SY, Harrington M, Chavasit V, Lynch SR, Hurrell RF. 2005. Comparison of the efficacy of wheat-based snacks fortified with ferrous sulfate, electrolytic iron, or hydrogen-reduced elemental iron: Randomized, double-blind, controlled trial in Thai women. *Am J Clin Nutr* 82:1276–1282.

A

Workshop Agenda

Dietary Reference Intake Research Synthesis
Workshop Agenda
June 7–8, 2006
The Keck Center of the National Academies
500 Fifth Street, NW, Room 100
Washington, DC 20001

Day 1—Wednesday, June 7
Moderators: John W Suttie and Susan J Whiting

8:30 a.m. Introductory Session
John W Erdman, Jr, PhD, University of Illinois—Urbana-Champaign
Paul M Coates, PhD, Office of Dietary Supplements, NIH, DHHS, Bethesda, MD
Peter Fischer, PhD, Bureau of Nutritional Sciences, Health Canada, Ottawa Canada
John W Erdman, Jr, PhD, University of Illinois—Urbana-Champaign

9:00 a.m. Database Session
Janice Rice Okita, PhD, RD, Institute of Medicine, Washington, DC

Discussion of Research Recommendations from the Nutrient Reports

9:30 a.m. DRIs for Calcium, Phosphorus, Magnesium, Vitamin D, and Fluoride
Bess Dawson-Hughes, MD, Tufts University, Boston, MA
Bruce W Hollis, PhD, Medical University of South Carolina, Charleston
Discussion

10:15 a.m. Break

10:30 a.m. DRIs for Thiamin, Riboflavin, Niacin, Vitamin B_6, Folate, Vitamin B_{12}, Pantothenic Acid, Biotin, and Choline
Steven H Zeisel, MD, PhD, University of North Carolina—Chapel Hill
Patrick J Stover, PhD, Cornell University, Ithaca, NY

11:15 a.m. DRIs for Vitamin C, Vitamin E, Selenium, and Carotenoids
Susan Taylor Mayne, PhD, Yale University School of Medicine, New Haven, CT
John N Hathcock, PhD, Council for Responsible Nutrition, Washington, DC
Discussion

12:00 p.m. Lunch Break

1:00 p.m. DRIs for Vitamin A, Vitamin K, Arsenic, Boron, Chromium, Copper, Iodine, Iron, Manganese, Molybdenum, Nickel, Silicon, Vanadium, and Zinc
Robert M Russell, MD, Tufts University, Boston, MA
Janet R Hunt, PhD, RD, USDA-ARS, Grand Forks Human Nutrition Research Center, Grand Forks, ND
Discussion

1:45 p.m. DRIs for Energy, Carbohydrate, Fiber, Fat, Fatty Acids, Cholesterol, Protein, and Amino Acids
Joanne R Lupton, PhD, Texas A&M University, College Station
Harold W (Bill) Kohl, III, PhD, Centers for Disease Control and Prevention, Atlanta, GA
Joanne L Slavin, PhD, RD, University of Minnesota, St Paul

2:45 p.m. DRIs for Water, Potassium, Sodium, Chloride, and Sulfate
Lawrence J Appel, MD, MPH, Johns Hopkins University, Baltimore, MD
Discussion

3:30 p.m. Break

Cross-Cutting Topics that Apply to Many Nutrients

3:45 p.m. New/Underutilized Research Techniques and the DRIs
Irwin H Rosenberg, MD, Tufts University, Boston, MA
Paul B Pencharz, PhD, MB, University of Toronto, ON, Canada
Jose M Ordovas, PhD, Tufts University, Boston, MA
Discussion

5:30 p.m. Adjourn for the Day

Day 2—Thursday, June 8
Moderators: John W Suttie and Susan J Whiting

Discussion of Research Recommendations from the Application Reports

8:30 a.m. DRIs: Applications in Dietary Assessment and Planning
Suzanne P Murphy, PhD, RD, University of Hawaii, Honolulu
Susan I Barr, PhD, RD, University of British Columbia, Vancouver, Canada
Jay Hirschman, MPH, Food and Nutrition Service, USDA, Alexandria, VA
Patricia M Guenther, PhD, RD, Center for Nutrition Policy and Promotion, USDA, Alexandria, VA
Rena Mendelson, DSc, RD, Ryerson University, Toronto, ON, Canada
Discussion

10:00 a.m. Break

Cross-Cutting Topics that Apply to Many Nutrients

10:15 a.m.	Setting DRIs for Children Lindsay H Allen, PhD, USDA, Western Human Nutrition Research Center, Davis, CA Nancy F Krebs, MD, University of Colorado Health Sciences Center, Denver Discussion
11:15 a.m.	Tolerable Upper Intake Levels (ULs) Sanford A Miller, PhD, University of Maryland—College Park Christine Taylor, PhD, Food and Drug Administration, Rockville, MD Discussion
12:00 p.m.	Wrap-up Session John W Suttie, PhD, University of Wisconsin, Madison Molly Kretsch, PhD, Agricultural Research Service, USDA, Beltsville, MD Hasan Hutchinson, PhD, ND, Institute of Nutrition, Metabolism and Diabetes, CIHR, Canada Catherine E Woteki, PhD, RD, Mars, Inc, McLean, VA Dennis M Bier, MD, Baylor College of Medicine, Houston, TX John Suttie, PhD, University of Wisconsin, Madison
1:00 p.m.	Adjourn Workshop

B

Workshop Presenters, Additional Participants, and U.S. and Canadian Government DRI Representatives

WORKSHOP PRESENTERS

Lindsay H. Allen, Ph.D.
United States Department of Agriculture
Western Human Nutrition Research Center, Davis, CA

Lawrence J. Appel, M.D., M.P.H.
Johns Hopkins University
Baltimore, MD

Susan I. Barr, Ph.D., R.D.
University of British Columbia
Vancouver, Canada

Dennis M. Bier, M.D.
Baylor College of Medicine
Houston, TX

Paul M. Coates, Ph.D.
Office of Dietary Supplements
National Institutes of Health
Department of Health and Human Services
Bethesda, MD

Bess Dawson-Hughes, M.D.
Tufts University
Boston, MA

John W. Erdman, Jr., Ph.D.
University of Illinois
Urbana-Champaign, IL

Peter Fischer, Ph.D.
Bureau of Nutritional Sciences
Health Canada, Ottawa, Canada

Patricia M. Guenther, Ph.D., R.D.
Center for Nutrition Policy and Promotion
United States Department of Agriculture, Alexandria, VA

John N. Hathcock, Ph.D.
Council for Responsible Nutrition
Washington, DC

Jay Hirschman, M.P.H.
Food and Nutrition Service
United States Department of Agriculture, Alexandria, VA

Bruce W. Hollis, Ph.D.
Medical University of South Carolina, Charleston, SC

Janet R. Hunt, Ph.D., R.D.
United States Department of Agriculture
Agricultural Research Service
Grand Forks Human Nutrition Research Center
Grand Forks, ND

Hasan Hutchinson, Ph.D., N.D.
Institute of Nutrition, Metabolism and Diabetes
Canadian Institutes of Health Research

Harold W. Kohl, III, Ph.D.
Centers for Disease Control and Prevention
Atlanta, GA

Nancy F. Krebs, M.D.
University of Colorado Health Sciences Center
Denver, CO

Molly Kretsch, Ph.D.
Agricultural Research Service
United States Department of Agriculture
Beltsville, MD

Joanne R. Lupton, Ph.D.
Texas A&M University
College Station, TX

Susan Taylor Mayne, Ph.D.
Yale University School of Medicine
New Haven, CT

Rena Mendelson, D.Sc., R.D.
Ryerson University
Toronto, ON, Canada

Sanford A. Miller, Ph.D.
University of Maryland
College Park, MD

Suzanne P. Murphy, Ph.D., R.D.
University of Hawaii
Honolulu, HI

Janice Rice Okita, Ph.D., R.D.
Institute of Medicine
Washington, DC

Jose M. Ordovas, Ph.D.
Tufts University
Boston, MA

Paul B. Pencharz, Ph.D., M.B.
University of Toronto
Ontario, Canada

Irwin H. Rosenberg, M.D.
Tufts University
Boston, MA

Robert M. Russell, M.D.
Tufts University
Boston, MA

Joanne L. Slavin, Ph.D., R.D.
University of Minnesota
St Paul, MN

Patrick J. Stover, Ph.D.
Cornell University
Ithaca, NY

John W. Suttie, Ph.D.
University of Wisconsin
Madison, WI

Christine Taylor, Ph.D.
Food and Drug Administration
Rockville, MD

Catherine E. Woteki, Ph.D., R.D.
Mars, Inc.
McLean, VA

Steven H. Zeisel, M.D., Ph.D.
University of North Carolina
Chapel Hill, NC

ADDITIONAL PARTICIPANTS

Stefanie Beddingfield
United States Department of Agriculture

Leila Beker
Food and Drug Administration

Jennifer Bhide
Grocery Manufacturers Association

Judy Blatman
Council for Responsible Nutrition

Mary Brandt
Food and Drug Administration

Danielle Brule
Health Canada

Margaret Cheney
Health Canada

Rebecca Costello
National Institutes of Health

Cindy Davis
National Cancer Institute

Paraskevi Detopoulou
Harokopio University

Kevin Dodd
National Cancer Institute

Johanna Dwyer
National Institutes of Health

Robert Earl
Food Products Association

Nicola Edwards
American Dietetic Association

Kathleen Ellwood
Food and Drug Administration

Nancy Emenaker
National Cancer Institute

Eileen Ferruggiaro
United States Department of Agriculture

MRC Greenwood
University of California-Davis

Joanne Guthrie
United States Department of Agriculture

Hedi Haddada
Embassy of France

Mary Hager
American Dietetic Association

Constance Hardy
Food and Drug Administration

Virginia Hartmuller
National Cancer Institute

Marcia Howard
Consumer Healthcare Products Association

Wen Yen Juan
Center for Nutrition Policy and Promotion

Christine Kaefer
National Cancer Institute

David Klurfeld
United States Department of Agriculture

Kathleen Koehler
Department of Health and Human Services

Susan Krebs-Smith
National Cancer Institute

Connye Kuratko
Martek Biosciences

Dorothy Lagg
Masterfoods USA

Elyse Levine
N. Chapman Associates

Jean Lloyd
Department of Health and Human Services

Kathryn McMurry
Department of Health and Human Services

Holly McPeak
Department of Health and Human Services

Gert Meijer
Unilever

Judith Moreines
Wyeth Consumer Healthcare

Sarah Murphy
Department of Health and Human Services

Mary Frances Picciano
National Institutes of Health

Jill Reedy
National Cancer Institute

Leila Saldanha
NutrIQ LLC

Andrew Shao
Council for Responsible Nutrition

Kathleen Smith
Food and Nutrition Associates

Pamela Starke-Reed
National Institutes of Health

Allison Stevens
N. Chapman Associates

Christine Tenekjian
Food Products Association

Elaine Trujillo
National Institutes of Health

Paula Trumbo
Food and Drug Administration

Jennifer Weber
American Dietetic Association

Kathy Wiemer
General Mills, Inc.

Albert Yamada
International Fresh Produce Council

Essie Yamini
United States Department of Agriculture

Allison Yates
United States Department of Agriculture

U.S. AND CANADIAN GOVERNMENT REPRESENTATIVES

Federal DRI Steering Committee

Department of Health and Human Services

*Office of Disease Prevention and Health Promotion**

Kathryn McMurry, M.S. (Chair, Federal DRI Steering Committee), Kimberly Stitzel, M.S., R.D. (until September 2005), and Jennifer Weber, M.P.H., R.D. (until May 2005)

Administration on Aging

Jean Lloyd, Ph.D.

Centers for Disease Control and Prevention

Division of Nutrition and Physical Activity

Elizabeth Tohill, Ph.D.

National Center for Health Statistics

Clifford Johnson, M.S.P.H.

Food and Drug Administration

Paula Trumbo, Ph.D., and Barbara Schneeman, Ph.D.

National Institutes of Health

Division of Nutrition Research Coordination*

Van Hubbard, M.D., Ph.D., and Pamela Starke-Reed, Ph.D.

National Heart, Lung, and Blood Institute

Darla Danford, Sc.D.

National Cancer Institute

John Milner, Ph.D.

Office of Dietary Supplements*

Paul Coates, Ph.D. (Co-Chair, Research Synthesis Subcommittee), Rebecca Costello, Ph.D., and Elizabeth Yetley, Ph.D.

Department of Agriculture

*Agricultural Research Service**

Molly Kretsch, Ph.D. (Co-Chair, Research Synthesis Subcommittee), and David Klurfield, Ph.D.

Center for Nutrition Policy and Promotion

Essie Yamini, Ph.D.

Cooperative State Research, Education, and Extension Service

Susan Welsh, Ph.D.

Department of Agriculture (continued)

Economic Research Service

Joanne Guthrie, Ph.D., and Elizabeth Frazao, Ph.D.

Food and Nutrition Service

Jay Hirschman, M.P.H. and Anita Singh, Ph.D.

Department of Defense

USARIEM

COL Karl Friedl, Ph.D.

Canadian Representatives and Liaisons to Steering Committee

Health Canada

*Food Directorate, Bureau of Nutritional Sciences**

Peter Fischer, Ph.D., Mary L'Abbé, Ph.D., and Nora Lee, M.Sc.

Office of Nutrition Policy and Promotion

Danielle Brulé, Ph.D.

Canadian Institutes of Health Research

*Institute of Nutrition, Metabolism and Diabetes**

Hasan Hutchinson, Ph.D.

DRI Research Synthesis Project Subcommittee

Paul Coates, Ph.D. (Co-Chair)*
Molly Kretsch, Ph.D. (Co-Chair)*
Peter Fischer, Ph.D.*
Hasan Hutchinson, Ph.D.*
Kathryn McMurry, M.S.*
Pamela Starke-Reed, Ph.D.*
John Milner, Ph.D.
Rebecca Costello, Ph.D.*
COL Karl Friedl, Ph.D.

NOTE: Project sponsors are noted with an asterisk (*) and are also listed separately on page 2 of the report.

C

List of Research Recommendations

The following research recommendations were generated from the database and are listed by ID Code.

DRI RECOMMENDATIONS

ID No.	ID CODE	RECOMMENDATION	DESIGNATION
1	A.I.02	Epidemiological research that evaluates the impact of habitual (lifetime) nutrient intake on functional outcomes related to specific diseases is urgently needed in order to optimize nutrient recommendations.	Major Knowledge
2	A.I.03	Epidemiological research that evaluates the impact of habitual (lifetime) dietary calcium intake on peak bone mass and fracture risk is urgently needed in order to optimize calcium recommendations.	Major Knowledge
3	A.I.04	Epidemiological research that evaluates the impact of habitual (lifetime) dietary calcium intake on prostate cancer is urgently needed in order to optimize calcium recommendations.	Major Knowledge
4	A.I.05	Epidemiological research that evaluates the impact of habitual (lifetime) dietary calcium intake on renal stones is urgently needed in order to optimize calcium recommendations.	Major Knowledge
5	A.I.06	Epidemiological research that evaluates the impact of habitual (lifetime) exposure to fluoride from all sources on prevention of dental caries and risk of fluorosis is urgently needed in order to optimize fluoride recommendations.	Major Knowledge

ID No.	ID CODE	RECOMMENDATION	DESIGNATION
6	A.I.07	Epidemiological research that evaluates the role of habitual (lifetime) dietary magnesium intake in the development of hypertension, cardiovascular disease, and diabetes is urgently needed in order to optimize magnesium recommendations.	Major Knowledge
7	A.I.08	Research is needed to assess methods for determining individual risk of chronic disease risk of chronic disease outcomes so that associations with nutrient status can be better understood.	Major Knowledge
8	A.I.09	The potential relationship between allelic variation in the vitamin D receptor (VDR), bone vitamin D receptor (VDR), bone mineral density, and osteoporosis within and between population groups requires further elucidation in order to determine if VDR polymorphisms are a variable influencing life-long calcium intake needs.	Major Knowledge
9	A.I.10	For children ages 1 through 18 years, research is needed to evaluate the dietary intakes of the dietary intakes of calcium, phosphorus, magnesium, and vitamin D required to optimize bone mineral accretion, especially in relation to changing age ranges for the onset of puberty and growth spurts.	Major Knowledge
10	A.I.11	With respect to dietary intake needs for vitamin D, information is required by geographical and racial variables that reflect the mix of the Canadian and United States populations and the influence of sunscreens on intake requirements.	Major Knowledge
11	A.II.02	Calcium balance studies should be augmented with stable or radioactive tracers of calcium to estimate aspects of calcium homeostasis with changes in defined intakes (i.e., fractional absorption, bone calcium balance, and bone turnover rates).	Research Method
12	A.II.03	Adaptations to changes in the amount of dietary calcium should be followed within the same populations for short-term (2 months) to long-term (1 to 2 years) studies. Different experimental approaches will be needed to define the temporal response to changes in dietary calcium. Short-term studies may be conducted in a metabolic research unit whereas the longer-term studies will need to be carried out in confined populations (i.e., convalescent home patients) fed prescribed diets; human study cohorts followed carefully for years with frequent, thorough estimates of dietary intakes; or metabolic studies of individuals fed their usual diets who typically consume a wide range of calcium intakes. All studies should include a comprehensive evaluation of biochemical measures of bone mineral content or metabolism. Bone mineral content and density should be evaluated in long-term studies. Good surro-	Knowledge Gaps

ID No.	ID CODE	RECOMMENDATION	DESIGNATION
		gate markers of osteopenia could be used in epidemiological studies.	
13	A.II.04	Investigations should include assessment of the effect of ethnicity and osteoporosis and osteoporosis phenotype on the relationship between dietary calcium, desirable calcium retention, bone metabolism, and bone mineral content.	Knowledge Gaps
14	A.II.05	Investigations should include evaluation of the independent impact of diet, lifestyle (especially physical activity), and hormonal changes on the utilization of dietary calcium for bone deposition and growth in children and adolescents. These studies need to be done in populations for which the usual calcium intakes range from low to above adequate.	Knowledge Gaps
15	A.II.06	Investigations should include epidemiological studies of the interrelationships between calcium intake and fracture risk, osteoporosis, prostate cancer, and hypertension must be pursued to determine if calcium intake is an independent determinant of any of these health outcomes. Control of other factors potentially associated as other risk factors for these health problems is essential (for example, fat intake in relation to cancer and cardiovascular disease; weight bearing activity; and dietary components such as salt, protein, and caffeine in relation to osteoporosis). Such epidemiological studies need to be conducted in middle-aged as well as older adult men and women.	Major Knowledge
16	A.II.07	Carefully controlled studies are needed to determine the strength of the causal association between calcium intake vis-à-vis the intake of other nutrients and kidney stones in healthy individuals.	Knowledge Gaps
17	A.II.08	Because of their potential to increase the risk of mineral depletion in vulnerable populations, calcium–mineral interactions should be the subject of additional studies.	Knowledge Gaps
18	A.III.01	The model that relates absorbed phosphorus intake to serum phosphorus must be evaluated in clinical studies using oral phosphorus intakes, and investigated in children and adolescents as well as adults.	Major Knowledge
19	A.III.02	Bone mineral mass as a function of dietary phosphorus intake should be investigated at all stages of the life cycle.	Knowledge Gaps
20	A.III.03	The practical effect of phosphate-containing food additives on trace mineral status (iron, copper, and zinc) should be evaluated.	Knowledge Gaps
21	A.IV.02	Reliable data on population intakes of magnesium are required based on dietary	Major Knowledge

ID No.	ID CODE	RECOMMENDATION	DESIGNATION
		surveys that include estimates of intakes from food, water, and supplements in healthy populations in all life stages.	
22	A.IV.03	Biochemical indicators that provide an accurate and specific marker(s) of magnesium status must be investigated in order to assess their ability to predict functional outcomes that indicate adequate magnesium status over prolonged periods.	Major Knowledge
23	A.IV.04	Basic studies need to be initiated in healthy individuals, including experimental magnesium depletion studies that measure changes in various body magnesium pools.	Major Knowledge
24	A.IV.05	Investigations should be conducted to determine the most valid units to use in expressing estimates of magnesium requirements (body weight, fat-free mass, or total body unit).	Major Knowledge
25	A.IV.06	Magnesium balance studies might be one indicator utilized as a marker of magnesium status. In magnesium balance studies, strict adherence to criteria suggested (IOM. 1997. Dietary Reference Intakes for Calcium, Phosphorus, Magnesium, Vitamin D, and Fluoride. Washington, DC: National Academy Press. Chapter 6—Magnesium) would improve their application to dietary recommendations.	Research Method
26	A.IV.07	Investigations are needed to assess the interrelationships between dietary magnesium intakes, indicators of magnesium status, and possible health outcomes that may be affected by inadequate magnesium intakes. Possible health outcomes include hypertension, hyperlipidemia, atherosclerotic vascular disease, altered bone turnover, and osteoporosis.	Major Knowledge
27	A.IV.08	Based on the evidence of abnormal magnesium status and health outcomes [from research in Recommendation ID Code A.IV.07 (pg. 249)], intervention studies to improve magnesium status and to assess its impact on specific health outcomes would be appropriate. Possible health outcomes include hypertension, hyperlipidemia, atherosclerotic vascular disease, altered bone turnover, and osteoporosis.	Knowledge Gaps
28	A.IV.09	The toxicity of pharmacological doses of magnesium requires further investigation.	Knowledge Gaps
29	A.V.01	Research is needed to evaluate how geographical and racial variables (that reflect the mix of the Canadian and American population) affect vitamin D status at various levels of vitamin D intake throughout the lifespan.	Knowledge Gaps
30	A.V.02	Research is needed to evaluate the influence of sunscreens on vitamin D status.	Knowledge Gaps
31	A.V.03	Regarding puberty and adolescence, research is needed to evaluate the effect of	Knowledge Gaps

ID No.	ID CODE	RECOMMENDATION	DESIGNATION
		various intakes of vitamin D on circulating concentrations of 25-hydroxyvitamin D [25(OH)D] and 1,25-dihydroxyvitamin D [1,25(OH)2D] during winter at a time when no vitamin D comes from sunlight exposure. During this time, the body adapts by increasing the renal metabolism of 25-hydroxyvitamin D [25(OH)D] to 1,25-dihydroxyvitamin D [1,25(OH)2D] and the efficiency of intestinal calcium absorption, thereby satisfying the increased calcium requirement by the rapidly growing skeleton.	
32	A.V.04	It is very difficult to determine the reference values for vitamin D in healthy young adults aged 18 through 30 and 31 through 50 years in the absence of sunlight exposure because of their typically high involvement in outdoor activity and the unexplored contribution of sunlight to vitamin D stores. More studies are needed that evaluate various doses of vitamin D in young and middle-aged adults in the absence of sunlight exposure.	Knowledge Gaps
33	A.V.05	A major difficulty in determining how much vitamin D is adequate for the body's requirement is that a normal range for serum 25-hydroxyvitamin D [25(OH)D] is 25 to 137.5 nmol/liter (10 to 55 ng/ml) for all gender and life stage groups. However, there is evidence, especially in the elderly, that in order for the parathyroid hormone (PTH) to be at the optimum level, a 25-hydroxyvitamin D [25(OH)D] of 50 nmol/liter (20 ng/ml) or greater may be required. Therefore, more studies are needed to evaluate other parameters of calcium metabolism as they relate to vitamin D status including circulating concentrations of parathyroid hormone (PTH).	Knowledge Gaps
34	A.V.06	The development of methodologies to assess changes in body stores of vitamin D is needed to accurately assess requirements in the absence of exposure to sunlight. Such work would markedly assist in the estimation of reference values for all life stage groups.	Research Method
35	A.VI.01	Epidemiological studies (especially analytical studies) of the relationships among fluoride exposures from all major sources and the prevalence of dental caries and enamel fluorosis at specific life stages should continue for the purposes of detecting trends and determining the contribution of each source to the effects demonstrated.	Knowledge Gaps
36	A.VI.02	Epidemiological and basic laboratory studies should further refine our understanding of the effects of fluoride on the quality and biomechanical properties of bone and on the calcification of soft tissue.	Knowledge Gaps

ID No.	ID CODE	RECOMMENDATION	DESIGNATION
37	A.VI.03	Studies are needed to define the effects of metabolic and environmental variables on the absorption, excretion, retention, and biological effects of fluoride. Such variables would include the composition of the diet (for example, calcium content), acid-base balance, and the altitude of residence.	Knowledge Gaps
38	B.I.01	Because of the difference in the bioavailability of food folate and the monoglutamate form of folate, it is recommended that both food folate and folic acid be included in tables and databases of food composition and in reports of intake. That is, the content or intake of naturally occurring food folate should be reported separately from that of folate provided by fortified foods and supplements.	Research Method
39	B.I.02	To fill information gaps, studies designed specifically to estimate average requirements in apparently healthy humans should be conducted for some micronutrients.	Major Knowledge
39.1	B.I.02.a	See Recommendation ID Code B.I.02.	Null
39.2	B.I.02.b	See Recommendation ID Code B.I.02.	Null
40	B.I.03	To fill information gaps, studies designed to generate usable data on the micronutrient needs of infants, children, adolescents, the elderly, and pregnant and lactating women should be conducted. Studies should use graded levels of nutrient intake and a combination of response indices.	Major Knowledge
40.1	B.I.03.a	See Recommendation ID Code B.I.03.	Null
40.2	B.I.03.b	See Recommendation ID Code B.I.03.	Null
40.3	B.I.03.c	See Recommendation ID Code B.I.03	Null
40.4	B.I.03.d	See Recommendation ID Code B.I.03.	Null
40.5	B.I.03.e	See Recommendation ID Code B.I.03.	Null
41	B.I.04	To fill information gaps, appropriately designed studies to determine the role of selected micronutrients in reducing the risk of certain chronic diseases should be conducted.	Major Knowledge
41.1	B.I.04.a	See Recommendation ID Code B.I.04.	Null
41.2	B.I.04.b	See Recommendation ID Code B.I.04.	Null
42	B.I.05	To fill information gaps, appropriately designed studies to determine the role of choline in reducing the risk of certain chronic diseases should be conducted.	Major Knowledge
43	B.I.06	To fill information gaps, studies designed to detect adverse effects of chronic high intakes of selected micronutrients should be conducted.	Major Knowledge
43.1	B.I.06.a	See Recommendation ID Code B.I.06.	Null

ID No.	ID CODE	RECOMMENDATION	DESIGNATION
43.2	B.I.06.b	See Recommendation ID Code B.I.06.	Null
43.3	B.I.06.c	See Recommendation ID Code B.I.06.	Null
44	B.I.08	Conduct studies to provide the basic data for constructing risk curves and benefit curves across the exposures to food folate and to folate (folic acid) added to foods and taken as a supplement. Such studies would provide estimates of the risk of developing neural tube defects, vascular disease, and neurological complications in susceptible individuals consuming different amounts of folate. With the new U.S. regulations on the fortification of cereal grains with folate, it is now possible to investigate the health effects, both positive and negative, of folate fortification on folate intake and health status.	Major Knowledge
44.1	B.I.08.a	See Recommendation ID Code B.I.08.	Null
44.2	B.I.08.b	See Recommendation ID Code B.I.08.	Null
45	B.I.09	Conduct investigations of the magnitude of the effect of intake of folate, vitamin B6, vitamin B12, and related nutrients for preventing vascular disease and other chronic degenerative diseases. Possible mechanisms for the influence of genetic variation should also be investigated.	Major Knowledge
45.1	B.I.09.a	See Recommendation ID Code B.I.09.	Null
45.2	B.I.09.b	See Recommendation ID Code B.I.09.	Null
46	B.I.10	Conduct studies to overcome the methodological problems in the analysis of folate, including the development of sensitive and specific deficiency indicators and of practical, improved methods for analyzing the folate content of foods and determining its bioavailability.	Major Knowledge
47	B.I.11	Conduct studies to develop economical, sensitive, and specific methods to assess the prevalence, causes, and consequences of vitamin B12 malabsorption and deficiency and to prevent and treat these conditions. One reason these methods are especially needed is because it appears that vitamin B12 deficiency greatly increases the potential of folate to cause adverse effects.	Major Knowledge
47.1	B.I.11.a	See Recommendation ID Code B.I.11.	Null
48	B.I.12	Investigate how folate and related nutrients influence normal cellular differentiation and development, including embryogenesis and neoplastic transformation.	Major Knowledge
49	B.I.13	Investigate vitamin B12 requirements of the elderly and how they may be met. These investigations appear to be a priority from a public health perspective.	Major Knowledge

ID No.	ID CODE	RECOMMENDATION	DESIGNATION
49.1	B.I.13.a	See Recommendation ID Code B.I.13.	Null
50	B.I.14	Investigate whether the folate requirement varies substantially by trimester of pregnancy. These investigations appear to be a priority from a public health perspective.	Major Knowledge
50.1	B.I.14.a	See Recommendation ID Code B.I.14.	Null
50.2	B.I.14.b	See Recommendation ID Code B.I.14.	Major Knowledge
51	B.I.15	Develop indicators on which to base vitamin B6 requirements.	Major Knowledge
52	B.II.01	Priority should be given to studies useful for setting Estimated Average Requirements (EARs) for thiamin for children, adolescents, pregnant and lactating women, and the elderly. Future studies should be designed around the Estimated Average Requirement (EAR) paradigm, use graded levels of thiamin intake with clearly defined cutoff values for clinical adequacy and inadequacy, and be conducted for a sufficient duration. To do this, close attention should be given to the identification of indicators on which to base thiamin requirements.	Major Knowledge
53	B.II.02	If studies are designed to test high doses of thiamin for possible beneficial effects, the design should also provide for the careful investigation of possible adverse effects.	Research Method
54	B.III.01	Priority should be given to studies useful for setting Estimated Average Requirements (EARs) for riboflavin for children, adolescents, pregnant and lactating women, and the elderly. Future studies should be designed specifically around the Estimated Average Requirement (EAR) paradigm, use graded levels of riboflavin intake and clearly defined cutoff values for clinical adequacy and inadequacy, and be conducted for a sufficient duration.	Major Knowledge
55	B.III.02	Develop another functional test for riboflavin status to corroborate and augment the presently used flavin–adenine dinucleotide-dependent erythrocyte glutathione reductase (e.g., a test using a flavin mononucleotide-dependent erythrocyte enzyme such as the pyridoxine [pyridoxamine] 5′-phosphate oxidase).	Knowledge Gaps
56	B.III.03	Examine the effects of physical activity on the requirement for riboflavin.	Knowledge Gaps
57	B.IV.01	For niacin, data useful for setting the Estimated Average Requirement (EAR) for children, adolescents, pregnant women, and lactating women are scanty. To fill information gaps, additional research on niacin requirements is desired for children, adolescents, pregnant women, and lactating women.	Knowledge Gaps
58	B.IV.02	Priority should be given to investigation of the niacin requirement to satisfy nicoti-	Major Knowledge

ID No.	ID CODE	RECOMMENDATION	DESIGNATION
		namide adenine dinucleotide (NAD) needs for increased adenosine diphosphate (ADP) ribosylation resulting from oxidant–deoxyribonucleic acid (DNA) damage.	
59	B.IV.03	Priority should be given to development of sensitive and specific blood measures of niacin status. Current assessments of niacin status and requirement are based solely on urinary metabolite measures; measurements of plasma metabolites such as the 2-pyridone derivatives may be productive. Two recent experimental studies have suggested erythrocyte nicotinamide adenine dinucleotide (NAD) as a functional blood measure of niacin status [Fu CS, Swendseid ME, Jacob RA, McKee RW. 1989. Biochemical markers for assessment of niacin status in young men: Levels of erythrocyte niacin coenzymes and plasma tryptophan. J Nutr 119(12):1949-1955; Ribaya-Mercado J, Russell R, Rasmussen H, Crim M, Perrone-Petty G, Gershoff S. 1997. Effect of niacin status on gastrointestinal function and serum lipids. FASEB J 11:A179. Abstract.], but further work is needed in clinical populations.	Major Knowledge
60	B.V.01	Priority should be given to studies useful for setting Estimated Average Requirements (EARs) for vitamin B6 for children, adolescents, pregnant and lactating women, and the elderly. Future studies should be designed around the Estimated Average Requirement (EAR) paradigm, use graded levels of nutrient intake and clearly defined cutoff values for clinical adequacy and inadequacy, and be conducted for a sufficient duration. To do this, close attention should be given to the identification of indicators on which to base vitamin B6 requirements.	Major Knowledge
60.1	B.V.01.a	See Recommendation ID Code B.V.01.	Null
61	B.VI.01	Investigations should be conducted to determine the mechanisms and magnitude of relationships of folate intake with risk reduction for the occurrence of neural tube defects (NTDs) and vascular disease and the influence of related factors (including genetic polymorphism) on these relationships. Targeted intervention programs need a clearer understanding of the mechanisms by which adequate folate intake ensures normal embryogenesis and may reduce vascular disease risk.	Major Knowledge
62	B.VI.02	Investigations should be conducted to estimate folate requirements in high-risk groups for which data are limited and for which public health problems may result from deficiencies. These groups include children, adolescents, women of reproductive age (including pregnant women by trimester and lactating women), and the elderly. These studies should identify and use new folate status indicators that are	Major Knowledge

ID No.	ID CODE	RECOMMENDATION	DESIGNATION
		linked to metabolic function and traditional indices of folate status.	
63	B.VI.03	Develop more precise and reproducible methods of analysis for the estimation of both blood and food folate and for the estimation of folate bioavailability. Improved methods would allow for comparison of status indicators among laboratories, revision of the food folate databases, and improved estimation of how dietary requirements are influenced by the food matrix and the source of folate (food or synthetic).	Research Method
64	B.VI.04	Identify and quantify adverse effects of high intakes of folate. Further investigation is needed on the effect of increasing folate intake from supplements and fortified foods on the onset and progression of vitamin B12 deficiency.	Major Knowledge
65	B.VI.05	Determine the mechanisms by which maternal folate sufficiency reduces the occurrence of neural tube defect (NTD) in the infant, including the establishment of which genes are responsible for the heritability and folate-responsiveness of NTD.	Knowledge Gaps
66	B.VI.06	Determine the effect of folate fortification on folate intake and occurrence of neural tube defect (NTD) and vascular disease. With the new U.S. regulations on the fortification of cereal grains with folate, it is now possible to investigate the health effects, both positive and negative, of folate fortification on folate intake and health status.	Major Knowledge
66.1	B.VI.06.a	See Recommendation ID Code B.VI.06.	Null
67	B.VI.07	Determine whether folate status affects the risk of birth defects other than neural tube defect (NTD) and of chronic diseases other than vascular disease (e.g., cancer). With the new U.S. regulations on the fortification of cereal grains with folate, it is now possible to investigate the health effects, both positive and negative, of folate fortification on folate intake and health status.	Major Knowledge
67.1	B.VI.07.a	See Recommendation ID Code B.VI.07.	Null
68	B.VII.01	Investigate the prevalence of vitamin B12 deficiency as diagnosed by biochemical, neurological, or hematological abnormalities (e.g., methylmalonic acid and holotranscobalamin II).	Major Knowledge
69	B.VII.02	Develop improved, economical, and sensitive methods to detect vitamin B12 malabsorption and deficiency before adverse neurological and hematological changes occur.	Major Knowledge
70	B.VII.03	Develop effective methods to reduce the risk of suboptimal vitamin B12 status resulting from vitamin B12 malabsorption or vegetarian diets. For elderly persons	Major Knowledge

ID No.	ID CODE	RECOMMENDATION	DESIGNATION
		with food-bound malabsorption, research is needed on the form and amount of vitamin B12 that can normalize and maintain vitamin B12 stores. For vegetarians, information is needed about the absorption of vitamin B12 from dairy products, algae, and fortified food products.	
71	B.VII.04	Investigate the feasibility, potential benefits, and adverse effects of fortification of cereal grain foods with vitamin B12 considering stability, identity of any degradation products, and bioavailability for normal individuals and those who malabsorb protein-bound vitamin B12.	Knowledge Gaps
72	B.VII.05	Investigate the contribution of bacterial overgrowth to elevated serum methylmalonic acid, to determine the variability of this indicator of vitamin B12 status.	Knowledge Gaps
73	B.VIII.01	To fill information gaps, further investigations about pantothenic acid as a nutrient are needed. Information gaps include human requirements, intake, bioavailability, toxicity, and metabolic effects. Research to date has indicated little cause for concern about the adequacy of pantothenic acid intake for healthy people; deficiency states can be produced only by actively interfering with the absorption or bacterial production pantothenic acid.	Major Knowledge
73.1	B.VIII.01.a	See Recommendation ID Code B.VIII.01.	Null
73.2	B.VIII.01.b	See Recommendation ID Code B.VIII.01.	Null
74	B.VIII.02	Investigate pantothenic acid requirements of different age groups, especially infants, children, and the elderly.	Major Knowledge
75	B.VIII.03	Investigate bioavailability of pantothenic acid from different foods and mixed diets and of the extent to which synthesis by intestinal bacteria contributes to meeting the requirement.	Major Knowledge
76	B.VIII.04	Using newer methods, such as high-pressure liquid chromatography, analyze pantothenic acid in foods. At present, pantothenic acid intakes are not calculated in national surveys such as the Third National Health and Nutrition Examination Survey (NHANES III) because of a lack of information on the pantothenic acid content of foods.	Major Knowledge
77	B.VIII.05	To fill information gaps, expand the food composition databases used for the national surveys to include pantothenic acid. This would allow pantothenic acid intakes to be calculated in national surveys such as the Third National Health and Nutrition Examination Survey (NHANES III).	Research Method

ID No.	ID CODE	RECOMMENDATION	DESIGNATION
78	B.IX.01	There is a serious lack of data useful for setting Estimated Average Requirements (EARs) for biotin. Although the limited information seems to indicate that there is little cause for concern about the adequacy of biotin intake for healthy people, information on the human requirements, intake, bioavailability, toxicity, and metabolic effects of this compound is needed. Deficiency states can be produced only by actively interfering with the absorption or bacterial production of biotin.	Major Knowledge
78.1	B.IX.01.a	See Recommendation ID Code B.IX.01.	Null
78.2	B.IX.01.b	See Recommendation ID Code B.IX.01.	Null
79	B.X.01	To fill information gaps, investigations should be conducted to obtain sufficient human data to determine whether choline is essential in the human diet, how much choline is required if it is essential, and the public health impact of poor choline nutriture. Although choline can be formed in the human body from endogenous precursors, little is known about dietary intake and the relative amounts of choline derived from the diet and from endogenous synthesis. Additional information gaps include bioavailability, toxicity, and metabolic effects.	Major Knowledge
79.1	B.X.01.a	See Recommendation ID Code B.X.01.	Null
79.2	B.X.01.b	See Recommendation ID Code B.X.01.	Null
80	B.X.03	Investigate the effects of the use of graded levels of dietary intake of choline on parameters of health. This would include assessing plasma and tissue choline compounds and metabolites; plasma cholesterol and homocysteine concentrations; erythrocyte folate; and liver, renal, brain, and other organ function. Animal studies suggest that choline intake may affect long-term health.	Major Knowledge
80.1	B.X.03.a	See Recommendation ID Code B.X.03.	Null
81	B.X.04	Data on the composition of human food are needed for choline, phosphocholine, glycerophosphocholine, sphingomyelin, phosphatidylcholine, and betaine and the analytic sensitivity and specificity of methods for analysis of food composition need to be validated.	Research Method
82	B.X.05	Human studies on interrelationships among requirements for choline, methionine, folate, vitamin B6, and vitamin B12 to compare the homocysteine-lowering effects of combinations of these nutrients are needed.	Major Knowledge
83	B.X.06	Investigate the relative effectiveness of different choline-containing compounds in the diet in promoting health and determination of the sparing effect of endogenous	Knowledge Gaps

ID No.	ID CODE	RECOMMENDATION	DESIGNATION
		synthesis of choline. It will be important to conduct studies on the bioavailability of choline and choline compounds and on the rate of de novo synthesis of choline in vivo.	
84	B.X.07	Conduct studies using increasing levels of dietary intake of choline designed to assess toxicity for all organ systems, including heart, liver, brain and kidney; fishy body odor; and possible growth suppression in children from observational data and as determined by experimental studies in animal models.	Knowledge Gaps
85	B.XI.04	For many nutrients, further investigation should be conducted on the biochemical values that reflect abnormal function.	Major Knowledge
85.1	B.XI.04.a	See Recommendation ID Code B.XI.04.	Null
85.2	B.XI.04.b	See Recommendation ID Code B.XI.04.	Null
86	B.XI.05	For many of the B vitamins, further investigation should be conducted on the relationship of existing status indicators to clinical end points to allow their use for setting Estimated Average Requirements (EARs).	Major Knowledge
87	B.XI.06	For some of the B vitamins, new clinical end points of impaired function need to be identified and related to status indicators.	Knowledge Gaps
88	B.XI.07	The depletion–repletion research paradigms that are often used in studies of requirements, although not ideal, are still probably the best approach to determining vitamin requirements. However, these studies should be designed to meet three important criteria. See B.XI.07a, B.XI.07b, and B.XI.07c.	Research Method
88.1	B.XI.07.a	An indicator of vitamin status is needed for which a cutoff point has been identified, below (or above) which vitamin status is documented to be impaired. (In the case of folate, an erythrocyte level of 300 nmol/L [140 ng/mL] fits this criterion because lower levels are associated with megaloblastic changes in blood cells. In the case of vitamin B6 and several other B vitamins, however, there is little information relating levels of status indicators to functional sufficiency or insufficiency. Instead, the levels of indicators normally used to assess requirements are those exhibited by subjects on a baseline adequate diet—even though there is no information regarding whether this level of intake is greatly in excess of adequate, barely adequate, or deficient.) The amount needed for restoration of biochemical status indicators to baseline values is not necessarily equivalent to the requirement for the nutrient.	Research Method
88.2	B.XI.07.b	The depletion and repletion periods should be sufficiently long to allow a new	Research Method

ID No.	ID CODE	RECOMMENDATION	DESIGNATION
		steady state to be reached. This can be very problematic because turnover rates of total body content for B vitamins range from less than 1 to about 3 percent per day, which suggests that long periods are needed for equilibrium. In the case of erythrocyte folate, theoretically the erythrocytes have to turn over completely (approximately 90 days). Study design should allow for examination of the effects of initial status on response to maintenance or depletion and repletion.	
88.3	B.XI.07.c	Intakes used in repletion regimens should bracket the expected Estimated Average Requirement (EAR) intake to assess the EAR more accurately and to allow for a measure of variance. In addition, an accurate assessment of variance requires a sufficient number of subjects.	Research Method
89	B.XI.08	A relatively new and increasingly popular approach to determining requirements is kinetic modeling of body pools using steady state compartmental analyses. This approach is unlikely to supplant depletion–repletion studies because it has a number of drawbacks; for example, a number of assumptions that cannot be tested experimentally are often needed and estimates obtained for body pool sizes are inherently imprecise. Even if accurate assessments of body pool sizes were possible and were obtained, such information would be useful in setting a requirement only if the size of the bodypool at which functional deficiency occurs could be established. The amount of the nutrient needed for restoration of biochemical status indicators to baseline values is not necessarily equivalent to the requirement for the nutrient.	Research Method
89.1	B.XI.08.a	See Recommendation ID Code B.XI.08.	Null
89.2	B.XI.08.b	See Recommendation ID Code B.XI.08.	Null
89.3	B.XI.08.c	See Recommendation ID Code B.XI.08.	Null
89.4	B.XI.08.d	See Recommendation ID Code B.XI.08.	Null
90	B.XI.10	For some of the B vitamins, studies should examine whether the requirement varies substantially by trimester of pregnancy.	Major Knowledge
91	B.XI.18	A growing number of studies suggests that there are complex interrelationships among nutrients (e.g., vitamin B6, folate, vitamin B12 and perhaps choline, methionine, and riboflavin), but these are not well understood in relation to the maintenance of normal nutritional status and to the prevention of chronic degenerative disease. These interactions may affect the need for one or more of the nutrients.	Major Knowledge
92	B.XI.20	For folate research, there are serious gaps in analytical methodology for the analysis	Major Knowledge

ID No.	ID CODE	RECOMMENDATION	DESIGNATION
		of blood folate and for the analysis of folate content of food. For folate, as for some other micronutrients, there are serious limitations in the methods available to analyze laboratory values indicative of nutrient status and to determine the nutrient content of foods. These methodological limitations have slowed progress in conducting or interpreting studies of nutrient requirements for folate.	
93	B.XI.21	To fill major knowledge gaps, compare the bioavailability of food folate from mixed diets and of folate in the form of folic acid (from supplements or fortification) consumed with food. This research should include an examination of the mechanisms by which bioavailability is altered by food matrices.	Major Knowledge
94	B.XI.23	Major gaps in knowledge include the mechanisms by which maternal folate sufficiency reduces the occurrence of neural tube defect (NTD) in the infant (e.g., evaluation of whether increased NTD risk is due to folate deficiency or to the mode of action of folate sufficiency [does it act on mother, embryo, or both?]); the relative efficacy of food folate, folate added to food, and folate supplements in reducing neural tube defect (NTD) risk; the process, if any, by which folate influences the embryonic process of neurulation; and the genes that are responsible for the heritability and folate-responsiveness of neural tube defect (NTD). See B.XI.23.a.	Major Knowledge
94.1	B.XI.23.a	Genetic studies of the heritability and folate-responsiveness of neural tube defect (NTD) could include: (1) linkage analyses in suitable genetically homogeneous human populations to assess the etiologic relationship between neural tube defect (NTD) and a variety of genetic alterations (including the thermolabile variant of 5,10-methylenetetrahydrofolate reductase) and in the genes responsible for NTD in the curly tail mouse; (2) investigation of whether alterations in any of these genes produce neural tube defect (NTD) when induced in mouse models, yield folate-responsive NTD in mouse models, and provide suitable markers for assessing NTD risk in human populations; and (3) identification of an animal model for common human neural tube defect (NTDs) that is responsive to relevant levels of folate.	Major Knowledge
95	B.XI.31	For B vitamins and choline as a group, only a few studies have been conducted that were explicitly designed to address adverse effects of chronic high intake. To allow sufficient data for deriving Tolerable Upper Intake Levels (ULs), additional research is required on the adverse effects of B vitamins and choline.	Knowledge Gaps
95.1	B.XI.31.a	See Recommendation ID Code B.XI.31.	Null

ID No.	ID CODE	RECOMMENDATION	DESIGNATION
96	C.I.01	Because the various forms of vitamin E are not interconvertible and because plasma concentrations of alpha-tocopherol are dependent upon the affinity of the hepatic alpha-tocopherol transfer protein for the various forms, it is recommended that relative biological potencies of the various forms of vitamin E be reevaluated.	Major Knowledge
97	C.I.02	Until research is completed to reevaluate the relative biological potencies of the forms of vitamin E, the actual concentrations of each of the various vitamin E forms in food and biological samples should be reported separately, wherever possible.	Research Method
98	C.I.06	To fill information gaps, validated biomarkers to evaluate oxidative stress and the relationship between antioxidant intake and health and disease should be identified.	Major Knowledge
99	C.I.08	Conduct studies to provide the basic data for constructing risk curves and benefit curves across the exposures to dietary and supplemental intakes of vitamin C, vitamin E, selenium, and beta-carotene and other carotenoids. These studies should be followed by nested case-control studies to determine the relationship of the biomarkers of oxidative stress to chronic disease. Finally, full-scale intervention trials should be done to establish the preventive potential of a nutrient for chronic disease.	Major Knowledge
100	C.I.09	Conduct investigations of gender specificity of the metabolism and requirements for vitamin C, vitamin E, selenium, and beta-carotene and other carotenoids. For example, women and children with low intakes of selenium are at higher risk of Keshan disease than are men with similar intakes. Women are at higher risk of macular degeneration even at similar plasma concentrations of carotenoids.	Major Knowledge
100.1	C.I.09.a	See Recommendation ID Code C.I.09.	Null
101	C.I.10	Conduct studies to validate methods and possible models for estimating Dietary Reference Intakes (DRIs) in the absence of data for some life stage groups, such as children, pregnant and lactating women, and older adults.	Major Knowledge
102	C.I.11	Conduct research to determine the interactions and possible synergisms of vitamin C, vitamin E, selenium, and beta-carotene with each other, with other nutrients and food components, and with endogenous antioxidants. Multifactorial studies are needed to demonstrate in vivo actions as well as synergisms that have been shown to occur in vitro.	Major Knowledge
103	C.I.12	Conduct studies to develop economical, sensitive, and specific methods to assess the associations of vitamin C, vitamin E, selenium, and beta-carotene and other carotenoids with the causation, prevalence, prevention,	Major Knowledge

ID No.	ID CODE	RECOMMENDATION	DESIGNATION
		and treatment of specific viral infections or other infections.	
104	C.I.13	Conduct investigations of the magnitude and role of genetic polymorphisms in the mechanisms of actions of vitamin C, vitamin E, selenium, and beta-carotene and other carotenoids.	Major Knowledge
105	C.II.01	Knowledge of vitamin C intakes needed to fulfill specific functional roles of ascorbate is needed to allow more accurate and precise determinations of the individual and average population requirements of vitamin C.	Major Knowledge
106	C.II.02	Some current candidates for specific functional roles of ascorbate that could be used as functional measures include pathways related to collagen and carnitine metabolism, oxidative damage, and oral health indices; however, research on new functions of vitamin C is needed.	Major Knowledge
107	C.II.03	Determination of vitamin C requirements based on antioxidant functions will require development of more reliable tests for in vivo oxidative damage and further understanding of the interactions of ascorbate with other physiological antioxidants.	Research Method
108	C.II.04	A practical method for measuring the vitamin C body pool is needed as a standard of comparison against proposed functional measures and measures of health or disease end points.	Research Method
109	C.II.05	Since the requirements for children ages 1 through 18 years are extrapolated from the adult Estimated Average Requirements (EARs), it is critically important to conduct large-scale studies with children using state-of-the-art biomarkers to assess their vitamin C requirement.	Major Knowledge
110	C.II.06	Population studies on the relationship of vitamin C nutriture and chronic disease should focus more on individuals or populations who eat few fruits and vegetables and are marginally deficient in vitamin C.	Research Method
111	C.II.07	Attention also has to be given to methods for sorting out the effects of vitamin C intake from those of other dietary and lifestyle factors that may also affect disease risk.	Research Method
112	C.II.08	While the evidence of adverse effects due to intakes of vitamin C supplements is limited at this time to osmotic diarrhea and gastrointestinal disturbances which are self-limiting, the frequency of high intakes of vitamin C in the North American population warrants further investigation. The well known pro-oxidant effects of the iron–ascorbate couple in vitro suggest that further research be done on possible	Knowledge Gaps

ID No.	ID CODE	RECOMMENDATION	DESIGNATION
		related in vivo reactions—for example, during simultaneous supplement ingestion, iron overload, and inflammation or tissue trauma where non-protein-bound iron may be released.	
113	C.II.09	A small number of isolated reports raise concern that high vitamin C intakes during pregnancy may expose the fetus or neonate to risks of withdrawal symptoms, hemolysis, or oxidant damage. Further research is needed to confirm or refute these concerns.	Knowledge Gaps
114	C.III.01	Biomarkers are needed for use in assessment of vitamin E intake and vitamin E status. What are the determinants of plasma concentrations of alpha-tocopherol, and are these concentrations regulated? Are plasma alpha-tocopherol concentrations the best parameter for assessing adequate plasma vitamin E status in apparently healthy individuals? Does an alpha-tocopherol/lipid (e.g., total lipid, triacylglycerol, or cholesterol) ratio better reflect optimal plasma vitamin E status?	Major Knowledge
115	C.III.02	Since the Recommended Dietary Allowances (RDAs) for vitamin E for children ages 1 through 18 years are extrapolated from the adult RDAs, it is critically important to conduct large-scale studies with children using state-of-the-art biomarkers to assess their vitamin E requirements.	Major Knowledge
116	C.III.03	Validate dietary intake instruments to assess intake of vitamin E. This methodology requires identification of the specific fats and oils consumed, in addition to careful tabulation of all of the foods consumed, because the vitamin E content of various fats and oils differs widely and because vitamin E is widely distributed in many foods. Most individual foodstuffs consumed account for less than 1 percent of the daily intake of alpha-tocopherol. Calories are frequently underreported, as is dietary fat, and the form and quantity of fat consumed are unknown. Better methods for estimating vitamin E intakes are needed.	Research Method
116.1	C.III.03.a	See Recommendation ID Code C.III.03.	Null
117	C.III.04	Information on the relationship between oxidative stress and vitamin E status is needed. Some information is available about the dosage of vitamin E needed to achieve plasma levels that protect circulating low-density lipoprotein (LDL) from ex vivo oxidation. However, there are scant data on tissue levels of vitamin E at different levels of intake. Do the large doses that confer protection of circulating low density lipoprotein (LDL) also confer protection within tissues against lipid	Knowledge Gaps

ID No.	ID CODE	RECOMMENDATION	DESIGNATION
		peroxidation or other manifestations of reactive oxygen species generation? Are there markers of oxidative stress that can be related to vitamin E status?	
117.1	C.III.04.a	See Recommendation ID Code C.III.04.	Null
118	C.III.05	Information on the nutrient requirement, metabolism and kinetics of vitamin E is needed. (1) Can estimates of alpha-tocopherol requirements be made using stable isotopes? (2) Are balance studies feasible that measure intake and output of stable isotope-labeled vitamin E? (3) What are the tissue uptake and subcellular distributions of alpha-tocopherol in humans? (4) What is the mechanism by which these nutrients are taken up and regulated by the cells? (5) What is the turnover of alpha-tocopherol in various human tissues? (6) In which tissues is alpha-tocopherol degraded and how rapidly? (7) What are the major metabolic intermediates during degradation of alpha-tocopherol, and do they have biological function?	Knowledge Gaps
118.1	C.III.05.a	See Recommendation ID Code C.III.05.	Null
119	C.III.06	Determination of the effects of vitamin E intake on the prevention of chronic disease is needed. There is a great deal of suggestive or indirect evidence that vitamin E intakes above those that can reasonably be obtained from foods may confer health benefits. See C.III.06.a and C.III.06.b.	Knowledge Gaps
119.1	C.III.06.a	Before clinical intervention trials can be interpreted properly, more knowledge about the relationship of vitamin E dosage to level of protection, or level of protection to plasma cholesterol or lipoprotein levels, is needed.	Knowledge Gaps
119.2	C.III.06.b	Additional clinical trials are needed to test directly whether or not supplementation with vitamin E can reduce the risk of coronary heart disease. A number of trials are in progress evaluating vitamin E effects in well over 100,000 individuals. However, whether the results are positive or negative, additional studies will be needed. For example, if the results are negative, the question will arise of whether treatment was instituted early enough and whether even longer trials starting at an earlier age are necessary to test the hypothesis properly. If the results are positive, the issue of dosage will arise. Most of these studies are supplementing with more than 200 mg/day of alpha tocopherol, but this may be unnecessarily high. Again, if the results are positive, indicating that vitamin E does indeed offer protection, it will be important to determine if combinations of antioxidants in various dosages can further increase the beneficial effect.	Knowledge Gaps

ID No.	ID CODE	RECOMMENDATION	DESIGNATION
120	C.III.07	Possible interactions between cholesterol-lowering treatments and antioxidant treatments (such as vitamin E) should be studied to find the best algorithm for preventive management of chronic disease.	Knowledge Gaps
121	C.III.08	More information is needed on the mechanisms of vitamin E function. It is unknown whether vitamin E functions solely as a relatively nonspecific antioxidant compound or whether it has some very specific modes of action, for which the precise structure of alpha-tocopherol is required. The mechanisms for regulation of tissue alpha-tocopherol are unknown. In fact, it is not known whether they are regulated at all. The relatively uniform concentrations in tissues from different individuals suggest that there may be regulation, but this may reflect differences in fat concentration.	Knowledge Gaps
122	C.III.09	The existence of alpha-tocopherol binding proteins in tissues other than the liver is being investigated. Do differences in depletion rates among various tissues reflect the functions of other tissue alpha-tocopherol binding proteins?	Knowledge Gaps
123	C.III.10	More information is needed on the other forms of vitamin E. What is the biological potency of forms of vitamin E other than alpha-tocopherol in humans? Does gamma-tocopherol have a role in humans? Does it function to act as a nitric oxide scavenger? What is the metabolic fate of gamma-tocopherol in humans?	Knowledge Gaps
124	C.IV.01	Biomarkers for use in assessment of selenium status are needed to prevent selenium deficiency and selenium toxicity. The relationship of plasma selenoprotein concentrations to graded selenium intakes must be studied in a severely selenium-deficient population in order to establish a more precise dietary selenium requirement. Plasma selenium levels (and other measurements of the element) have to be carried out in subjects fed levels of selenium (both organic and inorganic forms) up to the Tolerable Upper Intake Level (UL). This could validate use of plasma selenium concentrations to assess high levels of selenium intake.	Major Knowledge
125	C.IV.02	Since the Recommended Dietary Allowances (RDAs) for selenium for children ages 1 through 18 years are extrapolated from the adult RDAs, it is critically important to conduct large-scale studies with children using state-of-the-art biomarkers to assess their selenium requirements.	Major Knowledge
126	C.IV.03	Selenium functions largely through selenoproteins. Although the functions of some selenoproteins are known, those of others are not. Moreover, there appear to be a	Knowledge Gaps

ID No.	ID CODE	RECOMMENDATION	DESIGNATION
		number of selenoproteins that have not yet been characterized. Therefore, the functions of known and new selenoproteins need to be determined.	
127	C.IV.04	At present the recommendation for selenium intake has been set at the amount needed to achieve a plateau of the plasma selenoprotein glutathione peroxidase. Most residents in Canada and the United States can reach this level of selenium intake with their usual diet, but residents of many regions of the world have lower selenium intakes. Research is needed to determine the health consequences of selenium intakes inadequate to allow full selenoprotein expression.	Knowledge Gaps
128	C.IV.05	Limited evidence has been presented that intakes of selenium greater than the amount needed to allow full expression of selenoproteins may have chemopreventive effects against cancer. Controlled intervention studies are needed to fully evaluate selenium as a cancer chemopreventive agent.	Knowledge Gaps
129	C.V.01	Beta-carotene and other carotenoids have been shown to modulate a variety of intermediate end points. However, studies validating that changes in an intermediate end point are predictive of changes in a health outcome are critically needed.	Major Knowledge
130	C.V.02	Macular pigment optical density (MPOD) is a promising intermediate marker for age-related macular degeneration (AMD), and could be useful in studies of carotenoid requirements. However, human studies validating this end point prospectively are needed, as are studies demonstrating that changes in MPOD are predictive of changes in risk of macular degeneration.	Knowledge Gaps
131	C.V.03	Studies are needed on the effects of long-term depletion of beta-carotene and subsequent repletion, with an evaluation of validated intermediate end points.	Knowledge Gaps
132	C.V.04	Significantly more research is needed on health effects of dietary carotenoids other than beta-carotene. Possible associations between lycopene and decreased prostate cancer risk, between lutein and zeaxanthin and lowered risk of age-related macular degeneration (AMD), and between alpha-carotene or lutein and various cancers have to be evaluated in additional observational studies, in animal models, and in human intervention trials, if justified. Studies should consider not only the other carotenoids, but also the cis-versus trans-configuration of the carotenoid.	Major Knowledge
132.1	C.V.04.a	See Recommendation ID Code C.V.04.	Null
133	C.V.05	Since the data from the human intervention trials of beta-carotene are contradictory, additional data are needed from intervention trials involving beta-carotene, several	Knowledge Gaps

ID No.	ID CODE	RECOMMENDATION	DESIGNATION
		of which are ongoing. An examination is needed of health effects in populations with varying baseline risk profiles and, in particular, of studies evaluating interventions in populations with poor baseline nutritional status. Post-trial follow-up of completed beta-carotene trials is also needed.	
134	C.V.06	Studies aimed at the identification of correlates of higher beta-carotene intake and plasma concentrations, which might help to explain the lower risks of cancer associated with carotene-rich diets, are needed.	Knowledge Gaps
135	C.V.07	Additional research is needed that targets putative mechanisms to explain a possible increase in lung cancer risk in heavy smokers taking high-dose beta-carotene supplements (animal studies, biochemical studies, and molecular studies). In particular, confirmation and extension of findings such as those of recent reports regarding lung metaplasia [Wang XD, Liu C, Bronson RT, Smith DE, Krinsky NI, Russell M. 1999. Retinoid signaling and activator protein-1 expression in ferrets given beta-carotene supplements and exposed to tobacco smoke. J Natl Cancer Inst 91(1):60-66.] and carotenoid oxidation products [Salgo MG, Cueto R, Winston GW, Pryor WA. 1999. beta-carotene and its oxidation products have different effects on microsome mediated binding of benzo[a]pyrene to DNA. Free Radic Biol Med 26(1-2):162-173.], and their relevance to cancer development in humans, are needed.	Knowledge Gaps
136	C.V.08	Surveys are needed that routinely assess and report dietary intakes of individual food carotenoids from large, representative population samples. Intakes from both foods and dietary supplements must be considered.	Research Method
137	C.V.09	Efforts should be directed toward evaluating equivalency and demonstrating efficacy of carotenoids in foods to meet vitamin A needs in vitamin A-deficient populations, in order to develop sustainable strategies to eradicate this worldwide public health problem.	Major Knowledge
137.1	C.V.09.a	See Recommendation ID Code C.V.09.	Null
138	C.VI.05	For many micronutrients, a priority should be the determination of the relationship of existing status indicators to clinical end points in the same subjects to determine if a correlation exists.	Major Knowledge
138.1	C.VI.05.a	See Recommendation ID Code C.VI.05.	Null
139	C.VI.06	For vitamin C, vitamin E, selenium, and carotenoids, investigate the relationship of existing status indicators to clinical end points in the same subjects to determine if a	Major Knowledge

ID No.	ID CODE	RECOMMENDATION	DESIGNATION
		correlation exists.	
140	C.VI.07	For some nutrients, either new clinical end points or intermediate end points of impaired function have to be identified and related to status indicators.	Major Knowledge
141	C.VI.08	For vitamin C, vitamin E, selenium, and carotenoids, either new clinical end points or intermediate end points of impaired function have to be identified and related to status indicators	Major Knowledge
142	C.VI.09	The depletion–repletion research paradigms that are often used in studies of requirements, although not ideal, are still probably the best approach to determining nutrient requirements. However, these studies should be designed to meet three important criteria. See C.VI.09a. C.VI.09b, and C.VI.09c.	Research Method
142.1	C.VI.09.a	An indicator of nutrient status is needed for which a cutoff point has been identified, below which nutrient status is documented to be impaired. (In the case of vitamin E, values are based on induced vitamin E deficiency and the correlation with hydrogen peroxide-induced hemolysis and plasma alpha-tocopherol concentrations, because there is little information relating levels of status indicators to functional sufficiency or insufficiency. Also with vitamin C, there is little information relating levels of status indicators to functional sufficiency or insufficiency, because dose-dependent absorption and renal regulation of ascorbate allow body conservation during low intakes and limitation of plasma levels at high intakes.).	Research Method
142.2	C.VI.09.b	The depletion and repletion periods should be sufficiently long to allow a new steady state to be reached. (This can be very problematic for vitamin C because biological half-life ranges from 8 to 40 days and is inversely related to ascorbate body pool. For beta-carotene and other carotenoids, no long-term depletion–repletion studies with validated intermediate end points exist.) Study design should allow examination of the effects of initial status on response to maintenance or depletion–repletion.	Research Method
142.3	C.VI.09.c	Repletion regimen intakes should bracket the expected Estimated Average Requirement (EAR) intake to assess the EAR more accurately and to allow for a measure of variance. In addition, an accurate assessment of variance requires a sufficient number of subjects.	Research Method
143	C.VI.12	To fill gaps in information on vitamin C, vitamin E, selenium, and carotenoids, studies should examine whether or not the requirement varies substantially by tri-	Major Knowledge

ID No.	ID CODE	RECOMMENDATION	DESIGNATION
		mester of pregnancy.	
144	C.VI.13	To fill gaps in information on the nutrient requirements for vitamin C, vitamin E, selenium, and carotenoids, additional information is needed for groups at increased risk for oxidative stress, especially those who smoke or who are subjected to second-hand smoke, athletes, and individuals living at high altitudes.	Major Knowledge
145	C.VI.15	To fill information gaps, investigations should be conducted to advance the understanding of the health effects of carotenoids. Emphasis should be placed on bioavailability, toxicity, and health effects of carotenoids, since little information is available apart from beta-carotene.	Major Knowledge
146	C.VI.16	The only known validated function for carotenoids in humans is to act as a source of vitamin A in the diet. To fill information gaps, investigate the relative contribution of dietary provitamin A carotenoids to vitamin A status.	Major Knowledge
147	C.VI.17	Research to date has indicated little cause for concern about the adequacy of vitamin E intake for apparently healthy people; deficiency states can be produced only as a result of genetic abnormalities in alpha-tocopherol transfer protein, as a result of various fat malabsorption syndromes, or as a result of protein–energy malnutrition. However, investigation of the prevalence of these genetic abnormalities is needed.	Major Knowledge
148	C.VI.18	Investigate the health effects of nutrient-nutrient interactions. A growing number of studies suggest that there are complex interrelationships among nutrients, particularly those involved in protecting against oxidation (e.g., vitamin C, vitamin E, and selenium), but these are not well understood in relation to the maintenance of normal nutritional status and to the prevention of chronic degenerative disease. These interactions may affect the intake level for one or more of the nutrients.	Major Knowledge
149	C.VI.20	Develop assays for routine analysis of carotenoids. Although the analytical methodology for serum carotenoid status is becoming routine, methods for the analysis of the major dietary carotenoids remain as a limiting methodological factor.	Research Method
150	C.VI.21	Investigate the bioavailability of the various isomers of vitamin E. Compare the biological potencies of the various forms of vitamin E in food; these investigations should include mixed diets (that is, diets containing both plant-derived and animal-derived foods). Examine the mechanisms by which bioavailability of various forms of vitamin E is altered by food matrices.	Major Knowledge

ID No.	ID CODE	RECOMMENDATION	DESIGNATION
151	C.VI.23	Validate dietary intake instruments to assess intake of the major carotenoids in food.	Research Method
152	C.VI.24	To fill serious gaps in knowledge, investigate the relationship of intakes of vitamin C, vitamin E, selenium, and beta-carotene and other carotenoids to the risk of coronary heart disease, cancer, and other chronic degenerative diseases. An imbalance in oxidant stress and defenses can lead to the formation and excretion of oxidized products of nucleic acids, lipids, and proteins, which may play a role in chronic disease. Although interest is high and numerous studies have been conducted, additional investigations are needed.	Major Knowledge
153	C.VI.29	Vitamin E is known to protect ex vivo low-density lipoprotein oxidation, whereas beta-carotene offers no protection. Questions to be answered include the following: (1) what are the tissue uptake and subcellular distributions of beta-carotene in humans; (2) what is the mechanism by which beta-carotene is taken up and regulated by the cells; (3) what is the turnover of beta-carotene in the various tissues; (4) in which tissues is beta-carotene degraded and how rapidly; and (5) what are the major metabolic intermediates during degradation of beta-carotene and do they have biological function?	Knowledge Gaps
154	C.VI.30	Additional randomized clinical trials are needed to test whether or not supplementation with vitamin C, vitamin E, selenium, and/or beta-carotene and other carotenoids can reduce the risk of chronic disease. A number of clinical intervention trials involving more than 100,000 people are in progress. However, whether the results are positive or negative, additional studies will be necessary. See C.VI.30a, C.VI.30b, C.VI.30c, C.VI.30d, and C.VI.30e.	Major Knowledge
154.1	C.VI.30.a	Additional randomized clinical trials are needed to test whether or not supplementation with vitamin C, vitamin E, selenium, and/or beta-carotene and other carotenoids can reduce the risk of chronic disease. A number of clinical intervention trials involving more than 100,000 people are in progress. However, whether the results are positive or negative, additional studies will be necessary. If the results of ongoing clinical trials are negative, indicating that antioxidants do not offer protection, the question will arise as to whether treatment was instituted early enough and whether even longer trials starting at an earlier age are needed to test the hypothesis properly.	Major Knowledge

ID No.	ID CODE	RECOMMENDATION	DESIGNATION
154.2	C.VI.30.b	Additional randomized clinical trials are needed to test whether or not supplementation with vitamin C, vitamin E, selenium, and/or beta-carotene and other carotenoids can reduce the risk of chronic disease. A number of clinical intervention trials involving more than 100,000 people are in progress. However, whether the results are positive or negative, additional studies will be necessary. If the results of ongoing clinical trials are positive, indicating that antioxidants do indeed offer protection, the relative importance of vitamin C, vitamin E, selenium, and beta-carotene will have to be sorted out, because they are being used in combination in several of the studies.	Major Knowledge
154.3	C.VI.30.c	Additional randomized clinical trials are needed to test whether or not supplementation with vitamin C, vitamin E, selenium, and/or beta-carotene and other carotenoids can reduce the risk of chronic disease. A number of clinical intervention trials involving more than 100,000 people are in progress. However, whether the results are positive or negative, additional studies will be necessary. If the results of ongoing clinical trials are positive, indicating that antioxidants do indeed offer protection, the issue of dose will arise. Most of these studies are using doses that may be unnecessarily high.	Major Knowledge
154.4	C.VI.30.d	Additional randomized clinical trials are needed to test whether or not supplementation with vitamin C, vitamin E, selenium, and/or beta-carotene and other carotenoids can reduce the risk of chronic disease. A number of clinical intervention trials involving more than 100,000 people are in progress. However, whether the results are positive or negative, additional studies will be necessary. If the results of ongoing clinical trials are positive, indicating that antioxidants do indeed offer protection, the questions of who should be treated, at what dosage, and at what age will have to be addressed, along with the impact of treatment on various subgroups (older adults, those who smoke, those with other chronic diseases such as diabetes, etc.).	Major Knowledge
154.5	C.VI.30.e	Additional randomized clinical trials are needed to test whether or not supplementation with vitamin C, vitamin E, selenium, and/or beta-carotene and other carotenoids can reduce the risk of chronic disease. A number of clinical intervention trials involving more than 100,000 people are in progress. However, whether the results are positive or negative, additional studies will be necessary. If the results of on-	Major Knowledge

ID No.	ID CODE	RECOMMENDATION	DESIGNATION
		going clinical trials are positive, indicating that antioxidants do indeed offer protection, it will be important to determine if combinations of antioxidants in various doses can further increase the beneficial effect.	
155	C.VI.32	In cancer prevention studies, conduct additional randomized trials with vitamin E supplementation to confirmation or refutation the unexpected result of the Alpha-Tocopherol, Beta-Carotene Cancer Prevention Study in Finnish men.	Major Knowledge
156	C.VI.33	Data on the potential for beta-carotene to increase lung cancer rates in smokers are conflicting. Conduct additional randomized trials with beta-carotene supplementation to help resolve this issue.	Major Knowledge
157	C.VI.34	Because of inconsistent data, a Tolerable Upper Intake Level (UL) could not be established for beta-carotene, and due to a lack of sufficient data, ULs could not be set for other carotenoids from food. Thus, research is needed concerning the Tolerable Upper Intake Levels (ULs) for the carotenoids.	Major Knowledge
157.1	C.VI.34.a	See Recommendation ID Code C.VI.34.	Null
158	C.VI.35	Investigate the adverse effects of vitamin C, vitamin E, and selenium.	Knowledge Gaps
158.1	C.VI.35.a	See Recommendation ID Code C.VI.35.	Null
159	D.I.01	To fill information gaps, the specific role of selected micronutrients in human health should be investigated.	Major Knowledge
160	D.I.06	Conduct studies to identify and further understand the functional (e.g., cognitive function, regulation of insulin, bone health, and immune function) and biochemical end points that reflect sufficient and insufficient body stores of vitamin A, vitamin K, arsenic, boron, chromium, copper, iodine, iron, manganese, molybdenum, nickel, silicon, vanadium, and zinc.	Major Knowledge
161	D.I.07	Conduct studies to further identify and quantify the effects of interactions between micronutrients and interactions between micronutrients and other food components, the food matrix, food processing, and life stage on micronutrient (vitamin A, vitamin K, chromium, copper, iron, and zinc) bioavailability and therefore dietary requirement.	Major Knowledge
162	D.I.08	Conduct studies to further investigate the roles of arsenic, boron, nickel, silicon, and vanadium in human health.	Major Knowledge
163	D.I.09	Conduct studies to investigate the impact of non-nutritional factors (e.g., body mass index [BMI], glucose intolerance, infection) on the biochemical indicators for	Major Knowledge

ID No.	ID CODE	RECOMMENDATION	DESIGNATION
		micronutrients currently measured by U.S. and Canadian nutritional surveys, such as for iron and vitamin A. An example of such an impact is the evidence from national survey data that suggests that body mass index (BMI) and plasma glucose concentration are positively correlated with indicators of iron status. Such non-nutritional factors may markedly affect the interpretation of the survey data for certain subpopulations where the prevalence of non-nutritional factors is high.	
163.1	D.I.09.a	See Recommendation ID Code D.I.09.	Null
164	D.II.01	Investigate effects of food matrices (e.g., carotenoids in milk and supplements) on the bioavailability of provitamin A carotenoids.	Knowledge Gaps
165	D.II.02	Investigate age-related differences in the bioavailability of vitamin A.	Knowledge Gaps
166	D.II.03	Define critical end points for population assessment for vitamin A and evaluation of their association with liver vitamin A stores.	Knowledge Gaps
167	D.II.04	Investigate the effect of dietary vitamin A and vitamin A status on turnover and utilization of vitamin A. Is there significant adaptation to low vitamin A intakes? Is vitamin A absorption increased in response to low vitamin A intake? Is catabolism upregulated as body stores increase?	Knowledge Gaps
168	D.II.05	Investigate the relationship of bioactive vitamin A indicators (e.g., retinoic acid) to dietary vitamin A intake.	Knowledge Gaps
169	D.II.06	Investigate effects of pregnancy and lactation on maternal vitamin A turnover.	Knowledge Gaps
170	D.II.07	Investigate the effect of the interaction of vitamin A with other nutrients and food processing on the bioavailability of vitamin A.	Knowledge Gaps
171	D.III.01	Conduct clinical studies of vitamin K supplementation aimed at elucidating the physiological significance of undercarboxylated osteocalcin; these studies should be designed so as to relate this indicator to overall bone health and integrity.	Knowledge Gaps
172	D.III.02	Investigate the function of all of the vitamin K-dependent proteins and their role in human physiology.	Knowledge Gaps
173	D.III.03	Investigate the possible role of vitamin K in promoting human health other than that mediated by the known Gla-containing vitamin K-dependent proteins.	Knowledge Gaps
174	D.III.04	Investigate further the bioavailability of dietary vitamin K.	Knowledge Gaps
175	D.IV.01	Conduct controlled studies with low dietary intakes of chromium less than 5 to 15 mcg chromium/1,000 kilocalories) to determine an Estimated Average Requirement (EAR).	Knowledge Gaps

ID No.	ID CODE	RECOMMENDATION	DESIGNATION
176	D.IV.02	Investigate chromium absorption, metabolism, and requirements during pregnancy and lactation.	Knowledge Gaps
177	D.IV.03	Generate information on variability in chromium concentration in the food and water supply.	Knowledge Gaps
178	D.IV.04	Develop and validate a useful clinical indicator to identify persons with marginal chromium status and investigate effects of physiological levels of chromium supplementation in these patients.	Knowledge Gaps
179	D.IV.05	Investigate possible relationships between chromium status and insulin resistance, impaired glucose tolerance, and type 2 diabetes.	Knowledge Gaps
180	D.IV.06	Monitor any adverse effects of self-supplementation with chromium.	Knowledge Gaps
181	D.IV.07	Any research using supplementation with large-doses of chromium should be designed as controlled studies to assess both potential beneficial and potential adverse effects of large-dose supplementation of chromium.	Research Method
182	D.V.01	Investigate the specific health risks associated with marginal copper deficiency.	Knowledge Gaps
183	D.V.02	Conduct investigations to define the adverse effects of chronic high copper consumption for establishing Tolerable Upper Intake Levels (ULs) and to evaluate the health effects of copper supplements.	Knowledge Gaps
184	D.V.03	Conduct investigations to determine the involvement of low and high copper intakes on neurological and cognitive function.	Knowledge Gaps
185	D.VI.01	Investigate the correlation of community iodine intake with autoimmune thyroid disease and papillary thyroid cancer.	Knowledge Gaps
186	D.VI.02	Continually monitor U.S. urinary iodine by the National Health and Nutrition Examination Survey (NHANES) and include data on thyroid size in children, determined by ultrasound.	Research Method
187	D.VI.03	Investigate the role of iodine in fibrocystic breast disease.	Knowledge Gaps
188	D.VI.04	Investigate iodine nutrition and immune response.	Knowledge Gaps
189	D.VI.05	Investigate iodine nutrition in relation to other nutrients, particularly vitamin A, iron, and selenium.	Knowledge Gaps
190	D.VI.06	Investigate the effects of iodine concentration in water purification.	Knowledge Gaps
191	D.VI.07	Conduct investigations to further standardize thyroid volume by ultrasound and urinary iodine excretion in areas with different iodine intake.	Knowledge Gaps
192	D.VII.01	Conduct investigations to determine the significance of high ferritin concentration	Knowledge Gaps

ID No.	ID CODE	RECOMMENDATION	DESIGNATION
		in blood.	
193	D.VII.02	Investigate the effect of iron absorption and dietary iron on phenotypic expressions in individuals with hereditary hemochromatosis.	Knowledge Gaps
194	D.VII.03	Conduct research to distinguish between hereditary hemochromatosis and iron overload.	Knowledge Gaps
195	D.VII.04	Conduct research to study the effect of limited iron intake during pregnancy on infant iron status during the first 6 months of life.	Knowledge Gaps
196	D.VII.05	Investigate the bioavailability of supplemental iron.	Knowledge Gaps
197	D.VII.06	Conduct research to foster concurrence on valid indicators for assessing the effect of iron deficiency anemia on cognitive development and function.	Knowledge Gaps
198	D.VII.07	Investigate the risk of cardiovascular disease for those with high stores of body iron.	Knowledge Gaps
199	D.VII.08	Investigate the relationship between high iron stores in men and the bioavailability of dietary iron and impaired regulation of iron balance.	Knowledge Gaps
200	D.VII.09	Investigate the relationship between iron consumption and oxidative cellular damage.	Knowledge Gaps
201	D.VII.10	Investigate integrative mechanisms of iron transporter proteins that influence gastrointestinal absorption in various dietary conditions and physiologic states.	Knowledge Gaps
202	D.VIII.01	Conduct investigations to identify functional indicators for manganese.	Knowledge Gaps
203	D.VIII.02	Conduct investigations to analyze the effects of graded levels of dietary manganese intake on leukocyte superoxide dismutase activity or another appropriate functional indicator to provide an appropriate basis for setting an Estimated Average Requirement (EAR).	Knowledge Gaps
204	D.IX.01	Investigate the bioavailability of molybdenum.	Knowledge Gaps
205	D.IX.02	Conduct investigations to gather further data to estimate an average requirement for molybdenum.	Knowledge Gaps
206	D.X.01	Investigate biomarkers of zinc status based on functional outcomes; these biomarkers may be gene products derived from zinc-influenced systems and may include transporter proteins that provide homeostatic regulation of zinc intake and cellular processing.	Knowledge Gaps
207	D.X.02	Investigate the relationship of oxidative stress to zinc status.	Knowledge Gaps
208	D.X.03	Zinc salts are used therapeutically for treatment of some medical problems, but how	Knowledge Gaps

ID No.	ID CODE	RECOMMENDATION	DESIGNATION
		this relates to daily dietary zinc intake is not clear. Investigation is needed in this area.	
209	D.X.04	Investigate the effectiveness and potential toxicity of zinc as a dietary supplement. On which systems should zinc's potential effectiveness be based? Which systems become dysfunctional with excessive zinc intake?	Knowledge Gaps
210	D.X.05	Investigate the role of zinc in the various processes of the immune system, particularly those related to T-cell function at marginal zinc status.	Knowledge Gaps
211	D.X.06	Conduct investigations to generate quantitative data on human zinc homeostasis under a wide range of dietary conditions and at all ages using recent advances in zinc stable isotope methodology; these metabolic studies need to be long-term.	Knowledge Gaps
212	D.X.07	Conduct investigations to quantify what happens to zinc homeostasis as zinc intakes and absorption are increased and decreased beyond the range typically seen until recently; these metabolic studies need to be long-term.	Knowledge Gaps
213	D.XI.01	Conduct investigations to delineate a better understanding of species differences in biotransformation of arsenic and the toxicity of arsenic.	Knowledge Gaps
214	D.XI.02	Investigate the role of arsenic in methyl metabolism and genetic expression.	Knowledge Gaps
215	D.XI.03	Identify a reliable indicator of arsenic status in humans.	Knowledge Gaps
216	D.XI.04	Because relatively low serum arsenic concentrations have been associated with vascular diseases and central nervous system injury, more systematic investigation of the possible role of arsenic in these disorders is needed.	Knowledge Gaps
217	D.XII.01	Investigate the relationship between dietary boron and vitamin D metabolism.	Knowledge Gaps
218	D.XII.02	Investigate whether boron influences the half-life of functional vitamin D metabolites.	Knowledge Gaps
219	D.XII.03	Investigate whether boron influences calcium metabolism as it relates to bone mineralization.	Knowledge Gaps
220	D.XII.04	Investigate the possible influence of boron on estrogen metabolism and function, particularly biological half-life, receptor–ligand interactions, and estrogen-inducible gene expression as related to bone mineral density.	Knowledge Gaps
221	D.XII.05	Investigate the possible role of boron in human neurophysiological and cognitive function in young as well as older populations; these investigations should include delineation of a biochemical or other physiological basis for the role of boron.	Knowledge Gaps
222	D.XIII.01	Conduct investigations to identify and clearly characterize a biochemical function	Major Knowledge

ID No.	ID CODE	RECOMMENDATION	DESIGNATION
		for nickel in humans.	
222.1	D.XIII.01.a	See Recommendation ID Code D.XIII.01.	Null
223	D.XIII.02	Conduct investigations to identify a reliable indicator of nickel status for use in future studies of nickel deficiency.	Knowledge Gaps
224	D.XIII.03	Investigate the possible role of nickel in vitamin B12 and folate metabolism.	Knowledge Gaps
225	D.XIII.04	Investigate whether nickel nutrition should be a concern for pregnant women or people at risk for cardiovascular disease.	Knowledge Gaps
226	D.XIV.01	Investigate the physiological role of silicon and how this role relates to human health.	Major Knowledge
226.1	D.XIV.01.a	See Recommendation ID Code D.XIV.01.	Null
227	D.XIV.02	Investigate the possible role of silicon in atherosclerosis, hypertension, several bone disorders, Alzheimer's disease, and other conditions common to the elderly because of the prevalence and cost of these disorders.	Knowledge Gaps
228	D.XIV.03	Conduct investigations to determine a reliable indicator of silicon status.	Knowledge Gaps
229	D.XV.01	Conduct investigations to determine the biochemical role of vanadium in both higher animals and humans.	Major Knowledge
229.1	D.XV.01.a	See Recommendation ID Code D.XV.01.	Null
230	D.XV.02	Conduct investigations to determine a reliable status indicator of vanadium for further work in humans.	Knowledge Gaps
231	D.XV.03	Investigate the efficacy and safety of the use of vanadium as a nutritional supplement.	Knowledge Gaps
232	D.XVI.05	For vitamin A, vitamin K, arsenic, boron, chromium, copper, iodine, iron, manganese, molybdenum, nickel, silicon, vanadium, and zinc, investigate the relationship of existing status indicators to clinical end points in the same subjects to determine if a correlation exists.	Major Knowledge
233	D.XVI.06	For some micronutrients, either new clinical end points or intermediate end points of impaired function have to be identified and related to status indicators.	Major Knowledge
234	D.XVI.07	For vitamin A, vitamin K, arsenic, boron, chromium, copper, iodine, iron, manganese, molybdenum, nickel, silicon, vanadium, and zinc, either new clinical end points or intermediate end points of impaired function have to be identified and related to status indicators.	Major Knowledge
235	D.XVI.08	The depletion–repletion research paradigms and balance studies, although not ideal,	Research Method

ID No.	ID CODE	RECOMMENDATION	DESIGNATION
		are still probably the best approach to determining requirements for many of the trace minerals. However, these studies should be designed to meet three important criteria. See D.XVI.08a, D.XVI.08b, and D.XVI.08c.	
235.1	D.XVI.08.a	An indicator of nutrient status is needed for which a cutoff point has been identified, below which nutrient status is documented to be impaired. (In the case of manganese, serum manganese concentrations appear to be sensitive to large variations in manganese intake; however, there is a lack of information to indicate that this indicator reflects manganese status.)	Research Method
235.2	D.XVI.08.b	The depletion and repletion periods and balance studies should be sufficiently long to allow a new steady state to be reached. (For iodine and chromium, long-term balance studies are lacking.) Study design should allow examination of the effects of initial status on response to maintenance or depletion–repletion.	Research Method
235.3	D.XVI.08.c	Repletion regimen intakes should bracket the expected Estimated Average Requirement (EAR) intake to assess the EAR more accurately and to allow for a measure of variance. In addition, an accurate assessment of variance requires a sufficient number of subjects.	Research Method
236	D.XVI.11	For some of the micronutrients reviewed [list reviewed includes vitamin A, vitamin K, arsenic, boron, chromium, copper, iodine, iron, manganese, molybdenum, nickel, silicon, vanadium, and zinc], studies should examine whether the requirement varies substantially by trimester of pregnancy.	Major Knowledge
237	D.XVI.12	Data are lacking about gender specificity of the metabolism and nutrient requirements for some of the micronutrients reviewed [list reviewed includes vitamin A, vitamin K, arsenic, boron, chromium, copper, iodine, iron, manganese, molybdenum, nickel, silicon, vanadium, and zinc].	Major Knowledge
238	D.XVI.13	More information is needed on the vitamin A activity of carotenoids from plant-derived foods and mixed meals, including meat. Field trials, studying the vitamin A efficacy of plant-derived foods, are needed in which preformed vitamin A (positive control) is used at a supplementation level equivalent to plant-derived food interventions. Assessment of the bioconversion and retinol molar equivalency ratio of carotenoids has mostly been conducted on single foods; these assessments should be conducted on a mixture of fruits and vegetables. Newer methods, such as stable isotopic methods, to evaluate the bioconversion of provitamin A carotenoids to	Major Knowledge

ID No.	ID CODE	RECOMMENDATION	DESIGNATION
		vitamin A are encouraged. With such data, more information can be obtained about the relative contribution of dietary provitamin A carotenoids and dietary preformed vitamin A to vitamin A nutrition.	
239	D.XVI.15	There is increasing evidence to suggest that the interaction between micronutrients [list reviewed includes vitamin A, vitamin K, arsenic, boron, chromium, copper, iodine, iron, manganese, molybdenum, nickel, silicon, vanadium, and zinc] and other food components affect micronutrient absorption and metabolic utilization (bioavailability), but these interactions are not well understood in relation to the maintenance of normal nutritional status. These interactions may affect the dietary requirement for one or more of the micronutrients.	Major Knowledge
240	D.XVI.16	To fill information gaps, further research is needed to evaluate the metabolic role of arsenic, boron, nickel, silicon, and vanadium in human health. There is evidence that the five trace minerals have a role in some physiological processes in some species. For boron, silicon, and vanadium, measurable responses of human subjects to variation in dietary intake have been demonstrated. However, the available data are not as extensive and the responses are not as consistently observed as they are for the other micronutrients.	Major Knowledge
241	D.XVI.17	For some micronutrients [list reviewed includes vitamin A, vitamin K, arsenic, boron, chromium, copper, iodine, iron, manganese, molybdenum, nickel, silicon, vanadium, and zinc], serious limitations exist in the methods available to analyze laboratory values indicative of micronutrient status, to determine the micronutrient content of foods, or both. Standardization of indicators in relation to functional outcome is also needed. These methodological limitations have slowed progress in conducting or interpreting studies of micronutrient requirements.	Major Knowledge
241.1	D.XVI.17.a	See Recommendation ID Code D.XVI.17.	Null
241.2	D.XVI.17.b	See Recommendation ID Code D.XVI.17.	Null
242	D.XVI.18	Serious limitations exist in the methods available to determine chromium content of foods. This methodological limitation has slowed progress in generating data on chromium intake in North America and nutrient requirements. Develop improved, expedient methods for measuring chromium in food samples.	Research Method
243	D.XVI.19	Research on iodine is seriously limited by the lack of standardization of indicators in relation to functional outcome. This methodological limitation has slowed pro-	Major Knowledge

ID No.	ID CODE	RECOMMENDATION	DESIGNATION
		gress in conducting or interpreting studies of nutrient requirements. Conduct studies to further standardize thyroid volume and urinary iodine excretion to varying levels of iodine consumption.	
244	D.XVI.20	Further studies are needed for identifying the best indicator for assessing the effect of iron deficiency anemia on cognitive development. These methodological limitations have slowed progress in conducting or interpreting studies of nutrient requirements.	Major Knowledge
245	D.XVI.21	Potential sources of error in self-reported intake data include underreporting of portion sizes and frequency of intake, omission of foods, and inaccuracies related to the use of food composition tables and databases. Develop an acceptable method for adjusting intakes based on underreporting.	Research Method
245.1	D.XVI.21.a	See Recommendation ID Code D.XVI.21.	Null
246	D.XVI.22	Research is needed on the relationships of micronutrient intake to chronic disease. There are major gaps in knowledge linking the intake of specific micronutrients and the prevention or retardation of certain chronic diseases common in North America. For some micronutrients Estimated Average Requirements (EARs) are based on indicators other than functional ones.	Major Knowledge
247	D.XVI.23	A number of studies have been conducted to evaluate the role of vitamin K in maintenance of bone health. Additional studies are needed to understand the role of vitamin K in the prevention and retardation of chronic diseases common in North America such as osteoporosis.	Major Knowledge
248	D.XVI.24	A number of studies have demonstrated a beneficial effect of chromium on insulin action and circulating glucose levels. Additional research is needed to relate the intake of chromium to the prevention and reversal of diabetes, a chronic disease common in North America.	Major Knowledge
249	D.XVI.25	When sufficient information was available, Estimated Average Requirements (EARs) were based on functional indicators. For some micronutrients functional indicators were not apparent and Estimated Average Requirements (EARs) were based on other types of indicators. Additional research is needed to identify functional indicators of nutrient requirements for these micronutrients.	Major Knowledge
250	D.XVI.30	Because of lack of sufficient data, a Tolerable Upper Intake Level (UL) could not be established for vitamin K, arsenic, chromium, and silicon. Thus, research is	Knowledge Gaps

ID No.	ID CODE	RECOMMENDATION	DESIGNATION
		needed concerning the Tolerable Upper Intake Levels (ULs) for vitamin K, arsenic, chromium, and silicon.	
251	D.XVI.31	There was a lack of data from humans to establish a Tolerable Upper Intake Level (UL) for boron, molybdenum, and vanadium, and therefore a UL was based on animal data. Thus, human research is needed concerning the Tolerable Upper Intake Levels (ULs) for boron, molybdenum, and vanadium.	Knowledge Gaps
252	E.I.01	To fill information gaps, studies designed specifically to estimate average requirements for fiber and fat in presumably healthy humans should be conducted.	Major Knowledge
253	E.I.02	To fill information gaps, studies designed to generate data on the needs of macronutrients of infants, children, adolescents, the elderly, and pregnant and lactating women should be conducted.	Major Knowledge
254	E.I.03	To fill information gaps, multidose, long-term studies to determine the role of specific macronutrients in reducing the risk of certain chronic diseases should be conducted.	Major Knowledge
255	E.I.04	To fill information gaps, studies designed to detect adverse effects of chronic high intakes of specific macronutrients should be conducted. There are major gaps in knowledge linking the intake of some macronutrients and the prevention and retardation of certain chronic diseases common in North America. Because the relationship between macronutrient intake and risk of chronic disease is a trend, it is difficult to ascertain the optimal range of intake for each macronutrient.	Major Knowledge
255.1	E.I.04.a	See Recommendation ID Code E.I.04.	Null
256	E.I.05	Conduct long-term, dose–response studies to help identify the requirement of individual macronutrients that are essential in the diet (e.g., indispensable amino acids and n-6 and n-3 polyunsaturated fats) for all life stage and gender groups. It is recognized that it is not possible to identify a defined intake level of fat for maintaining health and decreasing risk of disease; however, it is recognized that further information is needed to identify acceptable ranges of intake for fat, as well as for protein and carbohydrate that are based on prevention of chronic disease and maintaining health.	Major Knowledge
256.1	E.I.05.a	See Recommendation ID Code E.I.05.	Null
257	E.I.06	Conduct studies to further understand the beneficial roles of dietary fiber and functional fibers in human health.	Major Knowledge

ID No.	ID CODE	RECOMMENDATION	DESIGNATION
258	E.I.07	Conduct studies designed to determine protein and energy needs during pregnancy. Do requirements vary substantially by trimester of pregnancy?	Major Knowledge
258.1	E.I.07.a	See Recommendation ID Code E.I.07.	Null
259	E.I.08	Conduct investigations to gather information on the form, frequency, intensity, and duration of exercise and physical activity that is successful in managing body weight in both children and adults.	Major Knowledge
260	E.I.09	Conduct long-term studies on the role of glycemic response in preventing chronic diseases, such as diabetes and coronary heart disease, in healthy individuals.	Major Knowledge
261	E.I.10	Conduct studies to investigate the levels at which adverse effects occur with chronic high intakes of macronutrients (carbohydrate, fiber, protein, and total fat).	Major Knowledge
261.1	E.I.10.a	See Recommendation ID Code E.I.10.	Null
262	E.II.01	Expand the number of available doubly labeled water studies for the determination of total energy expenditure (TEE) in certain age and gender categories, particularly in young children 3 to 5 years of age, adolescent boys, and adult men and women 40 through 60 years of age.	Major Knowledge
262.1	E.II.01.a	See Recommendation ID Code E.II.01.	Null
263	E.II.02	Develop reliable methods to track dietary energy intakes in population groups.	Research Method
264	E.II.03	Identify biological markers of risk of excess weight gain in children and young adults.	Knowledge Gaps
265	E.II.04	Develop methods suitable for free-living population-based studies or develop applications to measure physical activity levels in order to classify children and adults into sedentary, low active, active, and very active levels of physical activity.	Research Method
266	E.II.05	Conduct additional studies to determine whether and which dietary composition patterns facilitate permanent weight loss in adults and children.	Knowledge Gaps
267	E.II.06	Develop practical, accurate means to assess body composition in populations.	Research Method
268	E.II.07	Conduct investigations to describe physical activity patterns consistent with normal health and development of children that are applicable across age, gender, and ethnic backgrounds.	Major Knowledge
268.1	E.II.07.a	See Recommendation ID Code E.II.07.	Null
269	E.II.08	Conduct investigations to explore factors affecting the energy intake required to satisfy nutrient requirements, including diet digestibility, viscosity, and energy and nutrient density.	Knowledge Gaps

ID No.	ID CODE	RECOMMENDATION	DESIGNATION
270	E.II.09	Conduct investigation to identify factors affecting the changes in total energy expenditure (TEE) during pregnancy. Do requirements vary substantially by trimester of pregnancy? Develop equations to predict the basal metabolic rate (BMR) throughout pregnancy to better predict the energy requirements of nonobese, overweight, and obese pregnant women.	Major Knowledge
270.1	E.II.09.a	See Recommendation ID Code E.II.09.	Null
271	E.II.10	More information is needed on the energy requirements of overweight and obese adults and children. It would be desirable for this additional total energy expenditure (TEE) information to be collected in studies that also document physical activity patterns, so that the relationship between activity and TEE can be further evaluated.	Major Knowledge
271.1	E.II.10.a	See Recommendation ID Code E.II.10.	Null
272	E.II.11	Conduct additional research on the extent to which energy expenditure changes when a hypocaloric diet is consumed, and whether dietary composition affects the extent of change in energy expenditure.	Knowledge Gaps
273	E.II.12	Identify dietary components, independent of energy, that could favorably affect body composition.	Knowledge Gaps
274	E.III.01	Conduct additional research to elucidate the metabolic and long-term health differences resulting from the ingestion of high versus low glycemic index carbohydrates using larger, diverse sample sizes and whole-food diets.	Knowledge Gaps
275	E.III.02	Conduct investigations to determine if the energy density approach to weight reduction is effective in the long-term.	Knowledge Gaps
276	E.III.03	Conduct experimental studies to determine whether there is a metabolic effect of sugars in enhancing energy expenditure or in suppressing fat intake at a fixed level of energy.	Knowledge Gaps
277	E.III.04	Conduct research to determine the effect of low glycemic index foods and low glycemic-load diets on serum lipids and other risk factors for chronic disease and complications, especially in high-risk groups.	Knowledge Gaps
278	E.IV.02	Evaluate the protective effect of fiber against colon cancer in subsets of the population by applying genotyping and phenotyping to those participating in fiber and colon cancer trials. There also needs to be increased validation of intermediate markers, such as polyp recurrence, and assessment of functional markers (e.g., fecal	Major Knowledge

ID No.	ID CODE	RECOMMENDATION	DESIGNATION
		bulk) and its relationship to these end points.	
279	E.IV.03	Conduct a dose–response study to determine the amount of fiber that needs to be ingested to promote optimum laxation so that this could form the basis for a recommendation for fiber intake and provide a basis for determining functional fibers.	Major Knowledge
280	E.IV.04	Attempt to relate changes in the colonic microflora due to fiber ingestion to functional end points (e.g., decreased irritable bowel syndrome, increased laxation).	Major Knowledge
281	E.IV.05	Conduct longer-term studies on low energy-dense food sources (high in dietary fiber) and satiety and weight control to see if switching to a higher fiber diet will help with weight maintenance or promote adherence to reduced calorie diets for weight reduction.	Major Knowledge
282	E.IV.06	Examine the relation between dietary fiber intake, energy intake, and long-term body weight in existing prospective epidemiological studies in addition to intervention studies.	Major Knowledge
283	E.IV.07	Conduct long-term studies on the effects of both viscous and whole-grain cereal fibers on coronary heart disease and diabetes risk factors studies.	Major Knowledge
284	E.V.01	Conduct studies that examine the effects of alterations in the level of total fat in the context of a low saturated fatty acid diet on blood lipid concentrations and glucose–insulin homeostasis in individuals with defined metabolic syndromes, such as type 1 and type 2 diabetes.	Knowledge Gaps
285	E.V.02	Conduct randomized and blinded long-term (greater than 1 year) studies on the effect of dietary fat versus carbohydrate on body fatness.	Knowledge Gaps
286	E.V.03	Conduct investigations to further examine intakes of saturated fats at which significant risk of chronic diseases can occur.	Knowledge Gaps
287	E.V.04	Examine the indicators for and risk of chronic disease at low levels of saturated fatty acid intake.	Knowledge Gaps
288	E.V.05	Conduct investigations to assess energy balance in free-living individuals who have implemented a diet high in monounsaturated fatty acids versus a diet lower in monounsaturated fatty acids (and higher in carbohydrate).	Knowledge Gaps
289	E.V.06	Investigate the effects of alterations in the level of monounsaturated fatty acid in the context of a low saturated fatty acid diet on blood lipid concentrations and glucose–insulin homeostasis in individuals with defined metabolic syndromes, such as type 1 and type 2 diabetes.	Knowledge Gaps

ID No.	ID CODE	RECOMMENDATION	DESIGNATION
290	E.V.07	Conduct studies to evaluate cardiovascular disease risk status and risk of other chronic diseases in individuals consuming a high monounsaturated fatty acid diet versus a diet lower in monounsaturated fatty acids (and higher in carbohydrate).	Knowledge Gaps
291	E.V.08	Conduct an evaluation of the nutritional adequacy and nutrient profile of free-living individuals following a self-selected high monounsaturated fatty acid.	Knowledge Gaps
292	E.V.09	Conduct studies that assess the effects of a high monounsaturated fatty acid diet on endothelial function and atherogenesis.	Knowledge Gaps
293	E.V.10	In metabolic and large observational studies, compare the benefits of alpha-linolenic acid, eicosapentaenoic acid (EPA), and docosahexaenoic acid (DHA) across a range of n-6 polyunsaturated fatty acid intakes.	Knowledge Gaps
294	E.V.11	Using good biomarkers for low density lipoprotein (LDL) oxidation and cancer susceptibility, assess the potential adverse effects of diets at levels of n-6 polyunsaturated fatty acids greater than 10 percent of energy.	Knowledge Gaps
295	E.V.12	Conduct studies that assess the effects of a high n-6 polyunsaturated fatty acid diet on markers of endothelial function and inflammation.	Knowledge Gaps
296	E.V.13	Conduct additional research to address the potentially important relationships between the amount of n-3 and n-6 fatty acids and glucose tolerance suggested by studies of fatty acid composition in affected individuals.	Knowledge Gaps
297	E.V.14	Conduct randomized clinical trials of EPA+DHA, EPA (eicosapentaenoic acid), and DHA (docosahexaenoic acid) to evaluate their impact on cancer (i.e., colon, breast, prostate). The use of biomarkers for cancer susceptibility may expedite such studies.	Knowledge Gaps
298	E.V.15	Conduct randomized clinical trials of EPA+DHA, EPA (eicosapentaenoic acid), and DHA (docosahexaenoic acid) in treatment of inflammatory disorders (e.g., Crohn's disease, arthritis, psoriasis, asthma) and infections.	Knowledge Gaps
299	E.V.16	Conduct studies of EPA+DHA, EPA (eicosapentaenoic acid), and DHA (docosahexaenoic acid) supplementation in the elderly to prevent degenerative diseases of the central nervous system and retina, such as dementia, age-related macular degeneration (AMD), and night blindness.	Knowledge Gaps
300	E.V.17	Develop a comprehensive database for the trans fatty acid content of the United States food supply; use such a database to determine trans fatty acid intakes in different age and socioeconomic groups.	Knowledge Gaps

ID No.	ID CODE	RECOMMENDATION	DESIGNATION
301	E.V.18	Assess major sources of trans fatty acids currently in the marketplace; develop alternates similar to those developed for foods high in saturated fatty acids.	Knowledge Gaps
302	E.V.19	Conduct studies that distinguish trans fatty acid isomers from plants and animals with respect to the relative impact on blood lipid and lipoprotein concentrations.	Knowledge Gaps
303	E.V.20	In light of the wide variability of trans fatty acid intakes within food categories, develop a biochemical marker for trans fatty acid intake, independent of self-reported intake data.	Knowledge Gaps
304	E.VI.01	Conduct studies to identify possible mechanisms whereby early nutritional experiences, such as dietary cholesterol, affect the atherosclerotic process in adults and the sensitive periods in development when this may occur.	Knowledge Gaps
305	E.VI.02	Investigate the molecular mechanisms that regulate absorption of dietary cholesterol.	Knowledge Gaps
306	E.VI.03	Delineate specific genetic variants that contribute to wide interindividual variation in LDL (low density lipoprotein) cholesterol response to dietary cholesterol.	Major Knowledge
306.1	E.VI.03.a	See Recommendation ID Code E.VI.03.	Null
307	E.VI.04	Delineate dietary and constitutional factors (that is, non-genetic factors) that contribute to the wide interindividual variation in LDL (low density lipoprotein) cholesterol response to dietary cholesterol.	Major Knowledge
307.1	E.VI.04.a	See Recommendation ID Code E.VI.04.	Null
308	E.VI.05	Conduct studies to better define the relation between dietary cholesterol intakes and LDL (low density lipoprotein) cholesterol concentrations over a broad range of cholesterol intakes, from very low to high.	Knowledge Gaps
309	E.VI.06	Investigate the relationship between dietary cholesterol intakes and body pools of cholesterol.	Knowledge Gaps
310	E.VII.01	Conduct research on high protein intakes (greater than 145 mg nitrogen/kg body weight/day) in relationship to positive nitrogen balance and requirement estimates, metabolic and possible toxic effects in children and adults, and pathways impacted by these high intakes.	Knowledge Gaps
311	E.VII.02	Generate additional data on indispensable amino acid requirements for infants, children, and adolescents.	Major Knowledge
311.1	E.VII.02.a	See Recommendation ID Code E.VII.02.	Null
312	E.VII.03	Conduct further studies on the additional needs for protein during pregnancy; in-	Major Knowledge

ID No.	ID CODE	RECOMMENDATION	DESIGNATION
		clude estimates of changes in efficiency of conversion of dietary protein for maintenance and tissue accretion. Do requirements vary substantially by trimester of pregnancy?	
312.1	E.VII.03.a	See Recommendation ID Code E.VII.03.	Null
313	E.VII.04	Validate new methods, other than nitrogen balance, to determine protein requirements, particularly in regard to long-term health.	Research Method
313.1	E.VII.04.a	See Recommendation ID Code E.VII.04.	Null
314	E.VII.05	Investigate the role of the gastrointestinal system in the metabolism of amino acids, the nature of the amino acid losses, and the extent of synthesis of indispensable amino acids.	Knowledge Gaps
315	E.VII.06	Investigate adaptation mechanisms at various intakes of protein.	Knowledge Gaps
316	E.VII.07	To fill information gaps, investigate protein requirements in the elderly at various ages. Currently the protein data in the elderly are sparse. Available data for the very elderly, namely those from 80 to 100 years of age, consists of only two or three adults in their early eighties.	Knowledge Gaps
317	E.VII.08	To fill information gaps, investigate adverse effects of high intakes of amino acids. Tolerable Upper Intake Levels (ULs) could not be established for any of the amino acids (some of which are known to result in toxic effects at high doses) due to insufficient data on dose–response relationships.	Major Knowledge
317.1	E.VII.08.a	See Recommendation ID Code E.VII.08.	Null
318	E.IX.01	To fill information gaps, investigate the effect of exercise (i.e., endurance, resistance, other), frequency, intensity, and duration on body fatness in young and elderly adults and children.	Knowledge Gaps
319	E.IX.02	To fill information gaps, investigate the effects of exercise on substrate utilization and the roles of various energy depots (liver glycogen, muscle glycogen, adipose triacylglycerol, intramuscular triacylglycerol) in exercise and recovery in children, adults, and the elderly.	Knowledge Gaps
320	E.IX.03	Investigate whether the timing of meals and exercise can be used to optimize changes in, or to maintain favorable body mass index (BMI) and body composition of moderately and very active individuals.	Knowledge Gaps
321	E.IX.04	Investigate whether there are dietary compositions that optimize accretion of lean tissue in growing children and physically active adults.	Knowledge Gaps

ID No.	ID CODE	RECOMMENDATION	DESIGNATION
322	E.IX.05	Identify the mechanisms by which acute and chronic physical activity change substrate utilization and body composition.	Knowledge Gaps
323	E.IX.06	Develop reliable, noninvasive, and clinically appropriate measurements of body composition, cardiovascular function, and physical fitness.	Knowledge Gaps
324	E.IX.07	Develop practical, yet reliable methods to assess habitual levels of physical activity.	Knowledge Gaps
325	E.X.03	To fill information gaps related to some of the macronutrients, investigations should be conducted on the biochemical values that reflect abnormal function.	Major Knowledge
326	E.X.04	For n-6 and n-3 polyunsaturated fatty acids, investigations should be conducted on the biochemical values that reflect abnormal function.	Major Knowledge
327	E.X.05	A priority should be to determine if there is a correlation between existing status indicators for macronutrients and clinical end points in the same subjects.	Major Knowledge
328	E.X.06	For some macronutrients, more data are needed using clinical end points or intermediate end points of impaired function to determine their requirements in regard to long-term health.	Major Knowledge
329	E.X.07	For indispensable amino acids more data are needed using clinical end points or intermediate end points of impaired function to determine their requirements in regard to long-term health.	Major Knowledge
330	E.X.08	For determining energy requirements, investigations should be conducted on the form, frequency, intensity, and duration of exercise that is consistent with a healthy body weight for all age groups.	Major Knowledge
331	E.X.09	Additional studies should be conducted using doubly labeled water studies for the determination of total energy expenditure (TEE) in certain life stage and gender categories.	Major Knowledge
332	E.X.10	Investigate the role of n-3 polyunsaturated fatty acids in the neurodevelopment of term infants.	Major Knowledge
333	E.X.11	Investigations of nutrient requirements should use graded levels of nutrient intake and a combination of response indexes.	Research Method
334	E.X.14	For some macronutrients, serious limitations exist in the methods available to analyze laboratory values indicative of energy balance and macronutrient status. These methodological limitations have slowed progress in conducting or interpreting studies of energy and macronutrient requirements.	Major Knowledge
335	E.X.15	Develop biological markers of risk of excess weight gain in children and young	Major Knowledge

ID No.	ID CODE	RECOMMENDATION	DESIGNATION
		adults and standardize and validate indicators in relation to functional outcome. Past methodological limitations have slowed progress in conducting or interpreting studies of energy and macronutrient requirements.	
336	E.X.16	To better understand the relationship between fiber and colon cancer, further validate intermediate markers (such as polyp recurrence) and functional markers (such as fecal bulk) of fiber intake. Past methodological limitations have slowed progress in conducting or interpreting studies of energy and macronutrient requirements.	Major Knowledge
337	E.X.18	Reliable methods to track dietary energy intakes of populations need to be developed.	Research Method
338	E.X.19	Food composition tables and databases need to be expanded and revised to allow for further understanding of the relationship between macronutrient intake and health.	Research Method
339	E.X.20	A comprehensive database for the trans fatty acid content and glycemic index of foods consumed in North America is needed.	Research Method
340	E.X.22	Long-term, multidose clinical trials are needed to ascertain, for instance, the optimal range of total, saturated, and unsaturated fatty acids intake to best prevent chronic diseases such as coronary heart disease, obesity, cancer and diabetes.	Major Knowledge
341	E.X.23	Dose–response studies are also needed to determine the intake level of fiber to promote optimum laxation. To resolve whether or not fiber is protective against colon cancer in individuals or a subset of individuals, genotyping and phenotyping of individuals in fiber/colon cancer trials is needed.	Major Knowledge
342	E.X.24	Long-term clinical trials are needed to further understand the role of glycemic index in the prevention of chronic disease.	Major Knowledge
343	E.X.25	For some nutrients, such as saturated fat, trans fat, and cholesterol, biochemical indicators of adverse effects can occur at very low intakes. Clinical research should be conducted to ascertain clearly defined intake levels at which an onset of relevant health risks (e.g., obesity, coronary heart disease, and diabetes) occurs.	Major Knowledge
343.1	E.X.25.a	See Recommendation ID Code E.X.25.	Null
343.2	E.X.25.b	See Recommendation ID Code E.X.25.	Null
344	E.X.27	There is some animal data to suggest that high intakes of n-6 polyunsaturated fatty acids can increase the risk of certain types of cancer. Investigate this effect in humans.	Major Knowledge

ID No.	ID CODE	RECOMMENDATION	DESIGNATION
345	E.X.28	Conduct research to identify intake levels at which adverse effects begin to occur with the chronic consumption of high levels of protein and of the long chain n-3 polyunsaturated fatty acids (eicosapentaenoic acid and docosahexaenoic acid).	Major Knowledge
346	E.X.29	To fill information gaps, studies designed specifically to estimate average requirements for macronutrients in presumably healthy humans should be conducted.	Major Knowledge
347	F.I.01	To fill information gaps, studies to generate data for estimating average requirements for electrolytes and water in presumably healthy humans should be conducted.	Major Knowledge
348	F.I.02	To fill information gaps, studies designed to generate evidence on the electrolyte and water needs of infants, children, adolescents, the elderly, and pregnant and lactating women should be conducted.	Major Knowledge
349	F.I.03	To fill information gaps, multidose trials to determine the effects of electrolyte and water intake on chronic diseases should be conducted.	Major Knowledge
350	F.I.04	There is a critical need for research on public health strategies that effectively reduce sodium intake and increase potassium intake in the general population.	Major Knowledge
350.1	F.I.04.a	See Recommendation ID Code F.I.04.	Null
351	F.II.01	Develop simple non- or minimally-invasive indexes of body hydration status (both hyperosmotic and isoosmotic).	Knowledge Gaps
352	F.II.02	Conduct controlled water balance studies in different subgroups of the population (i.e., children, elderly, and those with chronic illnesses) in different climatic conditions.	Knowledge Gaps
353	F.II.03	Develop capabilities to predict hourly and daily water requirements based on metabolic rate, climatic conditions, and clothing for different subgroups of the population.	Knowledge Gaps
354	F.II.04	Conduct studies in water consumption and retention patterns due to meal schedule and diet.	Knowledge Gaps
355	F.II.05	Validate estimates of total water intake, both from food and fluids, in large-scale surveys.	Knowledge Gaps
356	F.II.06	Conduct additional studies on the effects of water deficits on cognitive performance.	Knowledge Gaps
357	F.II.07	Investigate the effects of water deficits on the risk of accidents, particularly when combined with heat or other environmental stresses (e.g., hypoxia).	Knowledge Gaps

ID No.	ID CODE	RECOMMENDATION	DESIGNATION
358	F.II.08	Conduct investigations to better understanding of the relationship between body water deficits and heat stroke or cardiac arrest associated with intense physical activity.	Knowledge Gaps
359	F.II.09	Investigate the influence of hydration status on morbidity-associated fever and infection outcome.	Knowledge Gaps
360	F.II.10	Investigate the effects of hydration status and fluid intake on the occurrence of urinary tract infections. The effects of increased water intake as a means to prevent recurrent urinary tract infections could be tested in clinical trials.	Major Knowledge
360.1	F.II.10.a	See Recommendation ID Code F.II.10.	Null
360.2	F.II.10.b	See Recommendation ID Code F.II.10.	Null
361	F.II.11	Investigate the effects of hydration status and fluid intake on chronic diseases, such as kidney stones and gallstones (cholelithiasis), as well as the occurrence of specific cancers, including colon cancer and bladder cancer. The effects of increased water intake as a means to prevent recurrent kidney stones and urinary tract infections could be tested in clinical trials. The relationship between water intake and bladder cancer could be addressed in observational studies.	Major Knowledge
361.1	F.II.11.a	See Recommendation ID Code F.II.11.	Null
361.2	F.II.11.b	See Recommendation ID Code F.II.11.	Null
362	F.II.12	Investigate the effects of chronic overhydration, in the presence of adequate sodium intake, on health and cognitive ability.	Knowledge Gaps
363	F.II.13	Investigate the mechanistic effects by which dehydration can contribute to exertional heat injury and heat stroke.	Knowledge Gaps
364	F.III.01	Conduct dose–response trials testing the effects of different levels of potassium intake on blood pressure at different levels of sodium intake.	Knowledge Gaps
365	F.III.02	Conduct additional dose–response trials evaluating the effect of potassium on salt sensitivity in subgroups of the population that are salt sensitive (e.g., African Americans, older persons, and persons with hypertension, chronic kidney disease, or diabetes).	Knowledge Gaps
366	F.III.03	Conduct randomized clinical trials to compare the effect of different potassium salts on blood pressure and other outcomes at different levels of sodium intake.	Knowledge Gaps
367	F.III.04	Develop improved measurements and instruments that assess total potassium intake and total body potassium.	Research Method

ID No.	ID CODE	RECOMMENDATION	DESIGNATION
368	F.III.05	Conduct trials that test the efficacy of increased potassium intake (alone and in combination with reduced sodium intake) on preventing stroke. To the extent possible, dose–response clinical trials should be conducted.	Major Knowledge
368.1	F.III.05.a	See Recommendation ID Code F.III.05.	Null
368.2	F.III.05.b	See Recommendation ID Code F.III.05.	Null
369	F.III.06	Conduct trials that test the main and interactive effects of potassium and sodium intake on bone mineral density and, if feasible, bone fractures. To the extent possible, dose–response clinical trials should be conducted.	Major Knowledge
369.1	F.III.06.a	See Recommendation ID Code F.III.06.	Null
369.2	F.III.06.b	See Recommendation ID Code F.III.06.	Null
370	F.III.07	Conduct trials testing the main and interactive effects of sodium and potassium intake on the risk of kidney stones. To the extent possible, dose–response clinical trials should be conducted.	Major Knowledge
370.1	F.III.07.a	See Recommendation ID Code F.III.07.	Null
370.2	F.III.07.b	See Recommendation ID Code F.III.07.	Null
371	F.III.09	Conduct studies on the role of potassium intake during infancy and childhood on blood pressure later in life.	Major Knowledge
371.1	F.III.09.a	See Recommendation ID Code F.III.09.	Null
372	F.III.10	Conduct potassium balance studies during pregnancy.	Knowledge Gaps
373	F.III.11	Develop better estimates of potassium losses in sweat with various dietary, activity, and environmental conditions in diverse populations.	Knowledge Gaps
374	F.III.12	Develop food composition tables or databases for citrate and bicarbonate.	Research Method
375	F.III.14	Conduct trials to assess the effects of high potassium intake on serum potassium levels and blood pressure in the setting of early stages of renal insufficiency (with and without ACE [angiotensin converting enzyme] inhibitor therapy).	Knowledge Gaps
376	F.IV.02	Conduct a broad spectrum of research with the aim of facilitating changes in individual behavior toward salt consumption to achieve reduced sodium intakes for most individuals in the United States and Canada.	Knowledge Gaps
377	F.IV.03	Conduct research to develop reduced sodium food products that maintain flavor, texture, consumer acceptability, and low cost.	Knowledge Gaps
378	F.IV.06	Develop effective public health strategies to achieve and sustain reduced sodium intakes and increased potassium intakes in the general population, including behav-	Major Knowledge

ID No.	ID CODE	RECOMMENDATION	DESIGNATION
		ioral change studies in individuals and community-based intervention studies.	
378.1	F.IV.06.a	See Recommendation ID Code F.IV.06.	Null
379	F.IV.07	Develop alternative processing technologies to reduce the sodium content of foods, with a special emphasis on maintaining flavor, texture, consumer acceptability, safety, and low cost.	Major Knowledge
379.1	F.IV.07.a	See Recommendation ID Code F.IV.07.	Null
380	F.IV.08	Conduct a formal assessment of the feasibility of a large-scale, long-term clinical trial designed to assess the impact of sodium reduction on clinical cardiovascular outcomes. The results of this assessment should be published.	Major Knowledge
380.1	F.IV.08.a	See Recommendation ID Code F.IV.08.	Null
380.2	F.IV.08.b	See Recommendation ID Code F.IV.08.	Null
381	F.IV.09	Investigate the main and interactive effects of sodium and potassium intake on non-cardiovascular clinical outcomes, specifically bone mineral density, osteoporosis, and kidney disease progression. There is some evidence that increased dietary sodium intake and inadequate potassium intake increase urinary calcium excretion and affect calcium balance.	Major Knowledge
381.1	F.IV.09.a	See Recommendation ID Code F.IV.09.	Null
382	F.IV.10	Assess the genetic and dietary factors that affect salt sensitivity.	Knowledge Gaps
383	F.IV.11	Increased renin activity is a potential biochemical indicator of inadequate sodium intake. In predominantly short-term studies, a reduced sodium intake increased plasma renin activity, but the clinical relevance of increased plasma renin activity is uncertain. Studies should be conducted to investigate the clinical relevance of sodium-induced changes in plasma renin activity.	Major Knowledge
383.1	F.IV.11.a	See Recommendation ID Code F.IV.11.	Null
383.2	F.IV.11.b	See Recommendation ID Code F.IV.11.	Null
384	F.IV.12	Studies should be conducted to investigate the main and interactive effects of sodium and potassium intake on plasma renin activity.	Knowledge Gaps
385	F.IV.13	Increased insulin resistance is a potential biochemical indicator of inadequate sodium intake. Data were insufficient to determine whether chronic ingestion of sodium in clinically relevant ranges led to deterioration in insulin resistance. Studies should be conducted to investigate the main and interactive effects of sodium and potassium intake on insulin resistance and glucose intolerance.	Major Knowledge

ID No.	ID CODE	RECOMMENDATION	DESIGNATION
385.1	F.IV.13.a	See Recommendation ID Code F.IV.13.	Null
385.2	F.IV.13.b	See Recommendation ID Code F.IV.13.	Null
385.3	F.IV.13.c	See Recommendation ID Code F.IV.13.	Null
386	F.IV.14	Develop practical tools to measure intakes of sodium and potassium and to assess total body levels of sodium and potassium.	Research Method
386.1	F.IV.14.a	See Recommendation ID Code F.IV.14.	Null
387	F.IV.15	Develop practical tools to define and measure salt sensitivity.	Knowledge Gaps
388	F.IV.16	Conduct investigations to better characterize salt sensitivity as a phenotype and determination of its relationship to cardiovascular outcomes.	Knowledge Gaps
389	F.IV.17	Investigate the influence of sodium intake during infancy and childhood on blood pressure later in life.	Major Knowledge
389.1	F.IV.17.a	See Recommendation ID Code F.IV.17.	Null
390	F.IV.18	Investigate the main and interactive effects of sodium and potassium intake on the age-related rise in blood pressure.	Knowledge Gaps
391	F.IV.19	Conduct sodium and potassium balance studies to provide estimates of electrolyte loss (sweat concentrations and total sweat loss) by physical activity level, climatic conditions, and dietary electrolyte intake in broad populations.	Knowledge Gaps
392	F.IV.20	Conduct sodium and potassium balance studies during pregnancy.	Knowledge Gaps
393	F.V.01	Investigate the relationship of urinary sulfate as a marker of sulfate absorption in evaluating adverse effects due to high intakes of sulfate.	Knowledge Gaps
394	F.V.02	Investigate sulfate supplementation of low-cysteine food products (e.g., casein-based enteral formula) to determine if supplementation improves growth or nitrogen balance.	Knowledge Gaps
395	F.V.03	Investigate sulfate needs during pregnancy, particularly the sulfate requirements of the growing fetus.	Knowledge Gaps
396	F.V.04	For sulfate, there is no indicator (i.e., biomarker) of inadequate intake. Evaluate using 3'-phosphoadenosine-5'-phosphosulfate or other biomarkers to determine dietary sulfate sufficiency.	Major Knowledge
396.1	F.V.04.a	See Recommendation ID Code F.V.04.	Null
397	F.V.05	Conduct investigations to generate better data on the relationship of diarrhea to sulfate intake in infants.	Knowledge Gaps
398	F.V.06	Investigate the effects of acute versus chronic sulfate ingestion on diarrhea as well	Knowledge Gaps

ID No.	ID CODE	RECOMMENDATION	DESIGNATION
		as whether and at what point adaptation occurs.	
399	F.V.07	Conduct survey studies comparing high versus low sulfate water ingestion from public water supplies that appropriately control for other causes of intestinal disturbances.	Knowledge Gaps
400	F.V.08	Conduct studies to evaluate whether chronic exposure to high sulfur (both cystine and sulfate) ingestion predisposes individuals to ulcerative colitis. Investigate the role of hydrogen sulfide in the etiology of ulcerative colitis.	Knowledge Gaps
401	F.V.09	Assess the relationship between increased sulfate intake and risk of inflammatory bowel disease. Conduct studies to determine how much of the sulfate produced via turnover in metabolism reenters the bowel and thus may serve as an irritant or oxidant. The risk of inflammatory bowel disease might be addressed in the setting of a case-control study or possibly a large, prospective observational study.	Major Knowledge
401.1	F.V.09.a	See Recommendation ID Code F.V.09.	Null
401.2	F.V.09.b	See Recommendation ID Code F.V.09.	Null
402	F.V.10	Conduct absorption studies using acute and chronic sulfate doses.	Knowledge Gaps
403	F.V.11	Conduct analytical studies to determine sulfate, as well as total sulfur content, of foods.	Knowledge Gaps
404	F.VI.12	For water, plasma or serum osmolality is an acceptable indicator of hydration status; however, trials that rigorously control and test different levels of total water intake, rather than allowing ad libitum intakes, have not been performed. These studies should be performed.	Major Knowledge
405	F.VI.14	For water, potassium, and sodium, useful data are lacking for setting requirements for infants, children, adolescents, pregnant and lactating women, and the elderly. Studies to collect these data should be conducted.	Major Knowledge
406	F.VI.15	There is a paucity of data on the relationship of dietary sodium and potassium intakes early in life on blood pressure and markers of bone health during adulthood. Studies to collect these data should be conducted.	Major Knowledge
407	F.VI.16	For water, potassium, and sodium, useful data are lacking for setting requirements for infants, children, adolescents, pregnant and lactating women, and the elderly. For water, research studies commonly tested the effects of inadequate intake in men of military age, but not in broad populations. These types of studies should be conducted.	Major Knowledge

ID No.	ID CODE	RECOMMENDATION	DESIGNATION
408	F.VI.17	Develop improved methods for the accurate measurement of total body water and electrolytes in free-living persons.	Research Method
409	F.VI.18	Develop improved methods for the accurate measurement of dietary intake of water and electrolytes in free-living persons. Potential sources of error in self-reported intake data include underreporting of portion sizes and frequency of intake, omission of foods and beverages, and use of food composition tables and databases.	Research Method
410	F.VI.19	Food composition tables and databases need to be continuously updated and expanded to include new foods and beverages and reformulated products. Inclusion of water and electrolytes in food composition tables and databases is important.	Research Method
411	F.VI.20	Develop practical tools to estimate sodium intake. For several reasons, assessment of sodium intake is problematic. Substantial additions can occur post-processing. In fact, many diet collection methods do not collect information on the salt (sodium chloride) added during cooking or eating. More importantly, there is large day-to-day variation in sodium intake. The most accurate method to assess dietary sodium is to measure several timed urinary collections. However, this approach is cumbersome and prone to collection errors. Hence, practical tools to estimate sodium intake are needed.	Research Method
412	F.VI.22	There is some evidence that increased dietary sodium intake and inadequate potassium intake increase urinary calcium excretion and affect calcium balance; to fill in knowledge gaps, additional investigations of effects of sodium and potassium intake on subclinical and clinical outcomes, such as bone mineral density and osteoporosis, are needed.	Major Knowledge
413	F.VI.32	Conduct studies that test the effects of reduced sodium and increased potassium intake, alone and combined, on clinical outcomes (e.g., stroke, bone mineral density, and kidney stones). To the extent possible, clinical trials should be conducted. A formal assessment of the feasibility of a sodium reduction trial with clinical cardiovascular outcomes should be undertaken. In the absence of trials, methodologically rigorous observational studies that concomitantly collect electrolyte intake, other dietary information, and genetic information should be conducted. There is some evidence that increased dietary sodium intake and inadequate potassium intake increase urinary calcium excretion and affect calcium balance.	Major Knowledge
413.1	F.VI.32.a	See Recommendation ID Code F.VI.32.	Null

ID No.	ID CODE	RECOMMENDATION	DESIGNATION
414	F.VI.33	Conduct studies to assess the potential for increased potassium intake to mitigate the adverse consequences of excess sodium intake and, vice versa, the potential for a reduced sodium intake to mitigate the adverse consequences of inadequate potassium intake. Potential outcomes include blood pressure, salt sensitivity, bone demineralization, and decreased bone mineral density. There is some evidence that increased dietary sodium intake and inadequate potassium intake increase urinary calcium excretion and affect calcium balance.	Major Knowledge
414.1	F.VI.33.a	See Recommendation ID Code F.VI.33.	Null
415	F.VI.34	Conduct studies on the adverse effects of chronic, low-grade metabolic acidosis that results from an inadequate intake of potassium and its bicarbonate precursors. Potential clinical outcomes include decreased bone mineral density, osteoporosis, and kidney stones.	Major Knowledge
415.1	F.VI.34.a	See Recommendation ID Code F.VI.34.	
416	F.VI.35	Conduct water, sodium, and potassium balance studies that enroll broad populations and that vary climate and physical activity levels. Populations of particular interest are children, as well as older persons with chronic, but stable, illnesses.	Major Knowledge
417	G.I.04	To fill knowledge gaps, conduct further investigations and collect better data on requirements for nutrients currently with an Adequate Intake (AI) (for age groups older than infants). Additional applications are possible when data are sufficient to allow Adequate Intakes (AIs) to be replaced with Estimated Average Requirements (EARs) (and thus Recommended Dietary Allowances [RDAs] can be set). Estimated Average Requirements (EARs) (rather than Adequate Intakes [AIs]) present more possibilities for assessing individual and group prevalence of inadequacy.	Major Knowledge
417.1	G.I.04.a	See Recommendation ID Code G.I.04.	Null
417.2	G.I.04.b	See Recommendation ID Code G.I.04.	Null
418	G.I.05	For nutrients with an Adequate Intake (AI) for age groups older than infants (vitamin D, vitamin K, pantothenic acid, biotin, choline, calcium, chromium, fluoride, manganese, potassium, sodium, chloride, water, dietary fiber, linoleic acid, and alpha-linolenic acid), new research and better data that allow replacement of the Adequate Intakes (AIs) with Estimated Average Requirements (EARs) and Recommended Dietary Allowances (RDAs) will greatly aid the assessment of nutrient adequacy.	Major Knowledge

ID No.	ID CODE	RECOMMENDATION	DESIGNATION
419	G.I.06	Collect better information on the distribution of requirements so that the appropriate method for assessing the prevalence of inadequacy for groups can be determined (EAR [Estimated Average Requirement] cut-point method versus full probability approach).	Null
419.1	G.I.06.a	See Recommendation ID Code G.I.06.	Major Knowledge
420	G.I.07	Research should be undertaken to allow Tolerable Upper Intake Levels (ULs) to be set for all nutrients. Establishment of Tolerable Upper Intake Levels (ULs) provides an opportunity to evaluate the risk of adverse effects for individuals and populations, and is an extremely important step forward in assessing intakes. Research to allow ULs to be set should be undertaken in carefully controlled settings.	
420.1	G.I.07.a	See Recommendation ID Code G.I.07.	Null
420.2	G.I.07.b	See Recommendation ID Code G.I.07.	Null
421	G.I.08	Research should be undertaken to generate information on ways to identify and conceptualize the risk of exceeding the Tolerable Upper Intake Level (UL). Information on the distribution of adverse effects via dose-response data (i.e., risk curves) would allow greatly expanded applications of ULs, particularly for population groups.	Major Knowledge
421.1	G.I.08.a	See Recommendation ID Code G.I.08.	Null
421.2	G.I.08.b	See Recommendation ID Code G.I.08.	Null
422	G.I.10	Develop new initiatives and innovative methods for the estimation and management of bias (such as underreporting or overreporting of food intake) during analysis of dietary intake data. This is a very high priority area of investigation.	Research Method
422.1	G.I.10.a	See Recommendation ID Code G.I.10.	Null
423	G.I.11	Advances are needed in behavioral research to determine why people underreport food intake.	Major Knowledge
424	G.I.12	Following advances in behavioral research to determine why people underreport food intake, develop improved dietary data collection tools that would not trigger this behavior.	Research Method
425	G.I.13	Following advances in behavioral research to determine why people underreport food intake, derive statistical tools to correct the bias associated with this phenomenon.	Research Method
426	G.I.14	To enhance estimates of nutrient inadequacy and estimates of nutrient intakes above	Research Method

ID No.	ID CODE	RECOMMENDATION	DESIGNATION
		the Tolerable Upper Intake Levels (UL), better ways to quantify the intake of dietary supplements are needed. This information is relevant to the nutrient status of a large proportion of the population in the United States and Canada. Investigation of better methods of quantifying dietary supplement intakes is a high-priority research area.	
426.1	G.I.14.a	See Recommendation ID Code G.I.14.	Null
426.2	G.I.14.b	See Recommendation ID Code G.I.14.	Null
427	G.I.15	Food composition databases need to be updated to include the forms and units that are specified by the Dietary Reference Intakes (DRIs).	Research Method
428	G.I.16	Develop chemical methodology to facilitate analysis of various forms of certain nutrients (e.g., alpha-tocopherol versus gamma-tocopherol) to allow comparison to the Dietary Reference Intakes (DRIs).	Research Method
429	G.I.17	Investigate methods for developing standard errors for prevalence estimates (such as those associated with requirement estimates).	Research Method
430	G.I.20	Further research is needed to apply the recommended assessment methods to estimate differences in the prevalence of inadequacy between subgroups, after controlling for other factors that affect nutrient intake.	Major Knowledge
431	G.I.21	Investigate ways to assess the performance of methods to estimate prevalence of inadequacy.	Major Knowledge
432	G.I.22	Conduct detailed investigations of the effects of violating assumptions for the EAR (Estimated Average Requirement) cut-point method. These investigations would best be done using well-designed, well-planned, and well-implemented simulation studies. Results of such studies would permit identification of recommendations as to the best approach to be used in assessments for each nutrient and would provide an estimate of the expected bias in prevalence estimates when the conditions for application of the EAR cut-point method are not ideal. Assumptions in applying the EAR cut–point method include: (a) intakes and requirements are not correlated or exhibit only low correlation; (b) the distribution of requirements in the population is approximately symmetrical; and (c) the variability of intakes is larger than the variability of requirements.	Major Knowledge
432.1	G.I.22.a	See Recommendation ID Code G.I.22.	Null
432.2	G.I.22.b	See Recommendation ID Code G.I.22.	Null

ID No.	ID CODE	RECOMMENDATION	DESIGNATION
433	G.II.10	Research on the factors that can alter nutrient requirements or upper limits is needed to enable more accurate applications of the Dietary Reference Intakes (DRIs) to specific individuals and populations. Adjustment factors for considerations such as body size, physical activity, and intakes of energy and other nutrients may be appropriate but are often unknown.	Knowledge Gaps
434	G.II.16	Develop and maintain a database of dietary supplement composition. This is difficult due to the rapidly changing market; however, investigation of better methods of quantifying dietary supplement intakes is a high-priority research area. Intake distribution from dietary supplements usually cannot be adjusted because the current data do not permit the estimation of the day-to-day variability in dietary supplement intake.	Research Method
435	G.II.20	Enhance food composition databases to separate nutrients inherent in foods from those provided by fortification, particularly when intakes are compared to the Tolerable Upper Intake Level (UL) for nutrients such as niacin.	Research Method
436	G.II.21	Modify food composition databases to change the units of measurement to those specified by the Dietary Reference Intakes (DRIs) (e.g., dietary folate equivalents [DFEs], as suggested for folate; milligrams of alpha-tocopherol, as suggested for vitamin E in place of alpha-tocopherol equivalents; and new biological conversion rates for beta-carotene to vitamin A as suggested for retinol activity equivalents in place of retinol equivalents).	Research Method
436.1	G.II.21.a	See Recommendation ID Code G.II.21.	Null
436.2	G.II.21.b	See Recommendation ID Code G.II.21.	Null
436.3	G.II.21.c	See Recommendation ID Code G.II.21.	Null
437	G.II.23	Research is needed to permit calculation of the standard deviation of daily intake for each individual. It is well known that the standard deviation of daily intake is typically heterogeneous across individuals. Conduct research to devise methods to allow the adjustment of a pooled standard deviation estimate to better reflect an individual's daily variability in intakes.	Research Method
438	G.II.24	Conduct research to devise methods for quantitatively assessing individual intakes when the distribution of daily intakes is not symmetrical around the individual's usual intake. The approach for testing whether usual intake is greater than requirements (or greater than the Adequate Intake [AI] or less than the Tolerable Upper	Research Method

ID No.	ID CODE	RECOMMENDATION	DESIGNATION
		Intake Level [UL]) makes the critical assumption that daily intakes for an individual are normally distributed. No alternative methodology exists for the many instances in which this assumption is untenable.	
439	G.II.26	Investigate methods for developing standard deviations for prevalence estimates (sometimes referred to as the standard error of the estimate) for use in assessing dietary intakes of groups.	Research Method
440	G.II.29	Investigate methods for developing an estimate of the standard deviation for the prevalence of nutrient inadequacy for use in assessing dietary intakes of groups. This concept combines two sources of uncertainty, the standard deviation of the Estimated Average Requirement (EAR) and the standard deviation of the usual intake distribution.	Research Method
441	G.II.30	Conduct research on ways to better match the biomarkers used to set requirements with the effect of dietary intake on those same biomarkers.	Knowledge Gaps
442	G.II.31	Conduct research on the appropriate biochemical data to collect so that these data can be combined with dietary intake data in assessment. Biomarker and other biochemical data are usually too expensive, time-consuming, or both, to collect on large numbers of individuals. However, when this information is available, it can be used in combination with intake data to give a more accurate estimate of the probability of inadequacy.	Knowledge Gaps
443	G.II.35	Conduct research in how to estimate differences in the prevalence of inadequacy between subgroups, after controlling for other factors that also affect nutrient intake. For example, a possible approach to addressing this issue based on multiple regression analysis has been described [see IOM, 2000, Dietary Reference Intakes: Applications in Dietary Assessment, Chapter 7]. Research is needed to apply this approach to existing survey data sets such as the Continuing Survey of Food Intakes by Individuals (CSFII) and the National Health and Nutrition Examination Surveys (NHANES).	Knowledge Gaps
444	G.II.39	Develop a wider variety of software that can assist users of the Dietary Reference Intakes (DRIs) in correctly applying the recommended methods.	Research Method
445	G.II.40	Upgrade software used currently in dietary assessment to incorporate the recommended statistical methodology.	Research Method
446	H.I.02	Pilot test the proposed approaches to dietary planning to achieve a low group preva-	Major Knowledge

ID No.	ID CODE	RECOMMENDATION	DESIGNATION
		lence of inadequate nutrient intakes. Before large-scale implementation of these approaches, practical pilot testing will be useful to assess whether a low prevalence of inadequacy can be achieved while meeting other important goals (e.g., avoiding excessive consumption of energy, maintaining nutrient intakes below the Tolerable Upper Intake Level [UL], and avoiding unnecessary food waste).	
446.1	H.I.02.a	See Recommendation ID Code H.I.02.	Null
446.2	H.I.02.b	See Recommendation ID Code H.I.02.	Null
447	H.I.03	Determine how different nutrition interventions affect intake distributions. It cannot be assumed that an intervention designed to increase the intake of a nutrient will result in a simple upward shift in nutrient intakes without changing the shape of the intake distribution or the between-person variation in usual nutrient intake. Different types of nutritional interventions may have very different effects on both the magnitude and shape of the intake distribution. Examination and publication of intake distributions before and after an intervention, with a systematic collection of this type of data, would allow a more informed selection of methods for planning a dietary intervention.	Major Knowledge
447.1	H.I.03.a	See Recommendation ID Code H.I.03.	Null
448	H.I.04	Determine the intake distributions of specific population groups. Although data on dietary intakes may be available either from national population surveys or surveys of large groups, often such information has not been reported in a manner that facilitates the estimation of variations in the usual intake of individuals.	Major Knowledge
449	H.I.05	Determine the relationship between foods offered and nutrient intake in the context of group planning. Research is needed to determine how food offerings relate to food and nutrient intakes, and how the relationship between food offered and intake varies according to planning context.	Major Knowledge
450	H.I.06	Develop and evaluate dietary planning strategies for heterogeneous groups, including a nutrient-density approach to dietary planning. Research is needed to determine the practical usefulness of planning for a target nutrient density, determine if the applicability of the nutrient density approach is limited to situations with predetermined food allocations or restricted food choices (e.g., emergency relief rations), and determine if this approach would be practical in situations offering a wide variety of food choices, where the nutrient density is more dependent on food selection	Major Knowledge

ID No.	ID CODE	RECOMMENDATION	DESIGNATION
		than on total food access to meet energy needs.	
451	H.I.10	Review and, where necessary, revise existing food guides. Changes in recommended intakes of various nutrients, combined with rapid changes in the amount and number of nutrients and types of foods that are fortified (particularly in the United States), necessitate review of existing food guides and continuation of the periodic review of dietary guidance such as the Dietary Guidelines for Americans and Canada's Guidelines for Healthy Eating.	Major Knowledge
451.1	H.I.10.a	See Recommendation ID Code H.I.10.	Null
452	H.I.11	Develop technical tools for the professional. There is a need to develop analytical tools that support implementation of recommendations for using the Dietary Reference Intakes (DRIs) for professional dietary assessment and planning, as well as for general guidelines for professionals to evaluate such tools. Industry and academia should explore development and production of accurate and convenient tools, expanding on the availability and use of sophisticated hand-held calculators and computers and easy Internet access to a spectrum of data and software.	Major Knowledge
452.1	H.I.11.a	See Recommendation ID Code H.I.11.	Null
453	H.I.12	Communicate with and educate nutrition professionals about correct uses of the Dietary Reference Intakes (DRIs). For full implementation and use of the DRIs, communication strategies are needed to effectively educate nutrition professionals on how the DRI recommendations can be practically and effectively applied. There is a need to formally examine how to best integrate this information into the education of nutrition professionals.	Major Knowledge
453.1	H.I.12.a	See Recommendation ID Code H.I.12.	Null
454	H.I.13	Assess application of the Dietary Reference Intakes (DRIs) for food and supplement labeling. The DRIs provide updated nutrient intake recommendations with scientific justification and extensive documentation. For some nutrients (e.g., folate and vitamin B12), the need to evaluate appropriate labeling information in both the United States and Canada is recognized to convey the recommendation for synthetic sources. Developing and testing a labeling format that conveys the meaning and use of the Tolerable Upper Intake Level (UL) may be especially helpful to consumers.	Major Knowledge
454.1	H.I.13.a	See Recommendation ID Code H.I.13.	Null
455	H.I.14	Develop and evaluate food guides for group planning. Planning for groups to have a	Major Knowledge

ID No.	ID CODE	RECOMMENDATION	DESIGNATION
		low prevalence of inadequate dietary intakes involves methods different from those used in planning for a low risk of dietary inadequacy for individuals. However, in both cases, the emphasis should be on food sources of nutrients. In the United States food-based menu planning guides have long been part of specifications for professionals to use in planning the food offered in various nutrition programs such as the National School Lunch Program. Convenient-to-use, food-based guidelines for menu planning for specific groups should be developed to assist professionals in planning for a low group prevalence of inadequate or excessive intakes.	
455.1	H.I.14.a	See Recommendation ID Code H.I.14.	Null
455.2	H.I.14.b	See Recommendation ID Code H.I.14.	Null
456	H.I.18	Identify factors that can alter the upper intake levels that can be tolerated biologically. For example, the nutrient source (such as a dietary supplement) can affect the potential risk of nutrient intakes that exceed the Tolerable Upper Intake Level (UL).	Major Knowledge
456.1	H.I.18.a	See Recommendation ID Code H.I.18.	Null
457	H.II.08	For situations in which nutrient density approaches are deemed useful, further development of data and methods is needed to estimate the median and distribution associated with nutrient requirements when expressed as a proportion of energy, either by statistical derivation from the present Estimated Average Requirements (EARs), or as a goal for future revisions of the Dietary Reference Intakes (DRIs).	Knowledge Gaps
458	H.II.09	Conduct further research to determine how intake distributions for all nutrients are affected when plans for heterogeneous groups involve targeting the aggregate or average requirement of specific nutrients for all individuals within a group versus targeting the maximum individual requirement for the whole group. Develop criteria to determine when to apply each of these approaches based upon current knowledge used to derive the Estimated Average Requirements (EARs) and Tolerable Upper Intake Levels (ULs), studies of intake distributions, and the effects of interventions. These criteria should consider the impact of such goal setting on the food supply and resulting distribution of intakes.	Knowledge Gaps
459	H.II.26	Studies to evaluate nutrient requirements or adverse effects of nutrient intakes should provide individual data where possible to allow estimation of their distributions.	Knowledge Gaps

D

DRI Research Synthesis Database Overview and Sample Printout

DRI RESEARCH SYNTHESIS DATABASE OVERVIEW

The research recommendations from the following eight reports (Box D-1) on Dietary Reference Intakes (DRIs) have been entered into a database to provide ready access to this material.

Note that the database was derived from the DRI reports and does not contain new information. The database is in the form of a Microsoft[1] Access file and a Microsoft Excel file; both files are available on the IOM project website (www.iom.edu/DRIresearch2006). The Access file contains all the research recommendations in ways that are easily accessible; the database can be searched easily by experienced Access users. The Excel file contains all the research recommendations plus other information (see below), but the accessibility of this information is limited by the capabilities of Excel.

[1]Microsoft Corporate Headquarters, Redmond, WA.

BOX D-1
DRI Reports Included in the Database

A: IOM. 1997. *Dietary Reference Intakes for Calcium, Phosphorus, Magnesium, Vitamin D, and Fluoride.* Washington, DC: National Academy Press.

B: IOM. 1998. *Dietary Reference Intakes for Thiamin, Riboflavin, Niacin, Vitamin B6, Folate, Vitamin B12, Pantothenic Acid, Biotin, and Choline.* Washington, DC: National Academy Press.

C: IOM. 2000. *Dietary Reference Intakes for Vitamin C, Vitamin E, Selenium, and Carotenoids.* Washington, DC: National Academy Press.

D: IOM. 2001. *Dietary Reference Intakes for Vitamin A, Vitamin K, Arsenic, Boron, Chromium, Copper, Iodine, Iron, Manganese, Molybdenum, Nickel, Silicon, Vanadium, and Zinc.* Washington, DC: National Academy Press.

E: IOM. 2002/2005. *Dietary Reference Intakes for Energy, Carbohydrate, Fiber, Fat, Fatty Acids, Cholesterol, Protein, and Amino Acids.* Washington, DC: The National Academies Press.

F: IOM. 2005. *Dietary Reference Intakes for Water, Potassium, Sodium, Chloride, and Sulfate.* Washington, DC: The National Academies Press.

G: IOM. 2000. *Dietary Reference Intakes: Applications in Dietary Assessment.* Washington, DC: The National Academies Press.

H: IOM. 2003. *Dietary Reference Intakes: Applications in Dietary Planning.* Washington, DC: The National Academies Press.

Database Fields

- ID No—*corresponds to the numerical order of total database entries*
- ID Code—*a code for internal use that corresponds to the code given to each database entry; the letter refers to the report (see later section "DRI Reports Included in the Database"*
- **Recommendation**—*full text of research recommendation*
- **Designation**—*determination made from wording in report and/or organization of the report*
  - Major Knowledge Gaps—research recommendation (knowledge gap) in the volume's summary or whose wording indicated at least one of the following: it was critically needed, critically important, particularly needed, must, or

    should be explored, merit(s) attention, is/are required. Location at the beginning of a section was also considered.
  - Knowledge Gaps—other research recommendations
  - Research Methods
- Priority Source—*describes what text in the report led to the priority designation or the location of the recommendation in the report that led to the priority designation*
- Keywords—*main words from the text of the recommendation*
- MeSH[2] Terms
- Type of Rec (Type of Recommendation)—*determination made from the original text of the recommendation*
  - General Research Recommendation
  - Specific Research Recommendation
  - Research Method
- Notes
- Exact Wording of Text—*text pulled directly from original DRI report*
- Page—*page number where recommendation can be found in given DRI report*
- Report Citation—*citation of the relevant DRI report*
- ISSB—*corresponds to particular report on the National Academies Press (NAP) website*
- Location/URL—*link to exact page (full text) on the NAP website*

Downloading and Usage Instructions

1. Website: http://www.iom.edu/DRIresearch2006. Click on the link for DRI Research Synthesis Database (on the right-hand side of the screen).
2. On the DRI Research Synthesis Database screen: Save the files to your computer as follows: click each file; this takes you to a webpage for that file; click START DOWNLOAD; select the SAVE option; in the "Save As" pop-up window choose an appropriate place to save the files on your computer. You will probably want to save both the Access file (.mdb) and the Excel file (.xls). You may choose to download this Accompanying Text file (.pdf), as well.
3. If you wish to view the database using Access:

[2]Medical Subject Headings

- If you are an experienced Access user:
  - Open the Access file that you have just saved to your computer.
  - Under "Objects/Tables" open the DRI Recommendations table, which is the database. Then use the functions of Access to view the data. We have created common Queries and Reports that you may wish to view as described below.
  - If you come across a Research Recommendation ID Code that is not in the Access database, look in the DRI-Other Text tab in the Excel file as described below.
- If you are a novice Access user:
  - Open the Access File that you have just saved to your computer.
  - Under "Objects/Reports" you will see numerous lists we created for common queries. Open or print any of these lists to view the selected data. Since we created over 100 lists, you may wish to use the "Groups" function to view lists in specific categories. This is the easiest way to view database entries. To view all the research recommendations related to calcium, for example, click on the Report named "Calcium List;" to view all of the Major Knowledge Gaps related to calcium, click on the Report named "Calcium List, Major." For any list you can right-click and choose print, or double-click to open and view the list.

4. If you wish to view the database using Excel:

   - Open the Excel file that you have just saved to your computer.
   - The first tab (DRI Recommendations) is the database, and you can view the entries using the functions of Excel. Note that there is not a convenient way to print this tab using Excel, however the other tabs are designed to print easily. Access provides the best way to view and print the database entries as reports.

5. Special features of the database, accessible only through Excel in the current version:
   - **DRI-Other Text** tab includes any other text from the DRI Reports that pertains to the research recommendations but was not actually used as a research recommendation. At present, printing this information from the Excel file is limited to specific data fields.

- **Glossary (DRI Recommendations)** tab lists definitions of acronyms, words, and terms used in the DRI Recommendations tab.
- **Glossary (DRI Reports)** tab lists definitions of acronyms, words, and terms used in any of the eight DRI reports.
- **Keywords** tab lists the keywords that were used to categorize the research recommendations. This field affects how queries in Access categorize the research recommendations.
- **MeSH** tab lists some of the Medical Subject Headings terms that will be used to categorize the research recommendations. This field affects how queries in Access categorize the research recommendations.
- **Glossary (MeSH)** tab lists some definitions used in applying the MeSH terms.
- **Numbers** tab gives some data about the database. Some of this information is listed in Box D-2.

BOX D-2
Numbers of Dietary Reference Intakes Research Recommendations

Total number of research recommendations: 459
Number of records by designation

- Major knowledge gaps: 212 (46.2%)
- Knowledge gaps: 199 (43.4%)
- Research methods: 48 (10.4%)

Priority Setting

The DRI panels were charged with developing prioritized research agendas to address research needs in scientific areas related to the DRIs. These research recommendations were not intended to provide a basis for public policy decisions and should not be interpreted as priorities for federal funding of research, which must consider a wide range of research needs in many scientific areas.

The individual DRI panels were guided in the task of priority setting by the following text from each report.

A: The following major research areas are considered the highest priority in order to more accurately determine the DRIs for calcium, phosphorus, magnesium, vitamin D, and fluoride in future reports.

B: The Standing Committee on the Scientific Evaluation of Dietary Reference Intakes (DRI Committee) agreed to assign highest priority to research that has potential to prevent or retard human disease processes and to prevent deficiencies with functional consequences. In the judgment of the DRI Committee and its panel and subcommittees, highest priority should be given to research that has potential to prevent or retard human disease processes and to prevent deficiencies with functional consequences.

C: Highest priority is thus given to research that has potential to prevent or retard human disease processes and to prevent deficiencies with functional consequences.

D: Highest priority is given to research that has the potential to prevent or retard human disease processes and to prevent deficiencies with functional consequences.

E: Highest priority is given to research that has the potential to prevent or retard human disease processes and to prevent deficiencies with functional consequences.

F: Highest priority is given to research that has the potential to prevent or retard human disease processes and to prevent deficiencies with functional consequences.

SAMPLE PRINTOUT PRODUCED BY MICROSOFT ACCESS

A-DRI Report on Calcium and Related Nutrients, List of All Research Recommendations

List of all research recommendations from the DRI Report on Calcium and Related Nutrients (v3; version 3 of the database).

Designation	ID No	ID Code	RECOMMENDATION
Major Knowledge Gaps	1	A.I.02	Epidemiological research that evaluates the impact of habitual (lifetime) nutrient intake on functional outcomes related to specific diseases is urgently needed in order to optimize nutrient recommendations.
Major Knowledge Gaps	2	A.I.03	Epidemiological research that evaluates the impact of habitual (lifetime) dietary calcium intake on peak bone mass and fracture risk is urgently needed in order to optimize calcium recommendations.
Major Knowledge Gaps	3	A.I.04	Epidemiological research that evaluates the impact of habitual (lifetime) dietary calcium intake on prostate cancer is urgently needed in order to optimize calcium recommendations.

Major Knowledge Gaps	4	A.I.05	Epidemiological research that evaluates the impact of habitual (lifetime) dietary calcium intake on renal stones is urgently needed in order to optimize calcium recommendations.
Major Knowledge Gaps	5	A.I.06	Epidemiological research that evaluates the impact of habitual (lifetime) exposure to fluoride from all sources on prevention of dental caries and risk of fluorosis is urgently needed in order to optimize fluoride recommendations.
Major Knowledge Gaps	6	A.I.07	Epidemiological research that evaluates the role of habitual (lifetime) dietary magnesium intake in the development of hypertension, cardiovascular disease, and diabetes is urgently needed in order to optimize magnesium recommendations.
Major Knowledge Gaps	7	A.I.08	Research is needed to assess methods for determining individual risk of chronic disease outcomes so that associations with nutrient status can be better understood.
Major Knowledge Gaps	8	A.I.09	The potential relationship between allelic variation in the vitamin D receptor (VDR), bone mineral density, and osteoporosis within and between population groups requires further elucidation in order to determine if VDR polymorphisms are a variable influencing lifelong calcium intake needs.

Major Knowledge Gaps	9	A.I.10	For children ages 1 through 18 years, research is needed to evaluate the dietary intakes of calcium, phosphorus, magnesium, and vitamin D required to optimize bone mineral accretion, especially in relation to changing age ranges for the onset of puberty and growth spurts.
Major Knowledge Gaps	10	A.I.11	With respect to dietary intake needs for vitamin D, information is required by geographical and racial variables that reflect the mix of the Canadian and United States populations and the influence of sunscreens on intake requirements.
Major Knowledge Gaps	15	A.II.06	Investigations should include epidemiological studies of the interrelationships between calcium intake and fracture risk, osteoporosis, prostate cancer, and hypertension must be pursued to determine if calcium intake is an independent determinant of any of these health outcomes. Control of other factors potentially associated as other risk factors for these health problems is essential (for example, fat intake in relation to cancer and cardiovascular disease; weight-bearing activity; and dietary components such as salt, protein, and caffeine in relation to osteoporosis). Such epidemiological studies need to be conducted in middle-aged as well as older adult men and women.
Major Knowledge Gaps	18	A.III.01	The model that relates absorbed phosphorus intake to serum phosphorus must be evaluated in clinical studies using oral phosphorus intakes, and investigated in children and adolescents as well as adults.

Major Knowledge Gaps	21	A.IV.02	Reliable data on population intakes of magnesium are required based on dietary surveys that include estimates of intakes from food, water, and supplements in healthy populations in all life stages.
Major Knowledge Gaps	22	A.IV.03	Biochemical indicators that provide an accurate and specific marker(s) of magnesium status must be investigated in order to assess their ability to predict functional outcomes that indicate adequate magnesium status over prolonged periods.
Major Knowledge Gaps	23	A.IV.04	Basic studies need to be initiated in healthy individuals, including experimental magnesium depletion studies that measure changes in various body magnesium pools.
Major Knowledge Gaps	24	A.IV.05	Investigations should be conducted to determine the most valid units to use in expressing estimates of magnesium requirements (body weight, fat-free mass, or total body unit).
Major Knowledge Gaps	26	A.IV.07	Investigations are needed to assess the interrelationships between dietary magnesium intakes, indicators of magnesium status, and possible health outcomes that may be affected by inadequate magnesium intakes. Possible health outcomes include hypertension, hyperlipidemia, atherosclerotic vascular disease, altered bone turnover, and osteoporosis.

Knowledge Gaps	12	A.II.03	Adaptations to changes in the amount of dietary calcium should be followed within the same populations for short- (2 months) to long-term (1 to 2 years). Different experimental approaches are needed to define the temporal response to changes in dietary calcium. Short-term studies may be conducted in metabolic research units whereas the longer-term studies need to be carried out in confined populations (i.e., convalescent home patients) fed prescribed diets; human study cohorts followed for years with frequent, thorough estimates of dietary intakes; or metabolic studies of individuals fed their usual diets who typically consume a wide range of calcium intakes. All studies should include a comprehensive evaluation of biochemical measures of bone mineral content or metabolism. Bone mineral content and density should be evaluated in long-term studies. Good surrogate markers of osteopenia could be used in epidemiologic studies.
Knowledge Gaps	13	A.II.04	Investigations should include assessment of the effect of ethnicity and osteoporosis phenotype on the relationship between dietary calcium, desirable calcium retention, bone metabolism, and bone mineral content.
Knowledge Gaps	14	A.II.05	Investigations should include evaluation of the independent impact of diet, lifestyle (especially physical activity), and hormonal changes on the utilization of dietary calcium for bone deposition and growth in children and adolescents. These studies need to be done in populations for which the usual calcium intakes range from low to above adequate.

Knowledge Gaps	16	A.II.07	Carefully controlled studies are needed to determine the strength of the causal association between calcium intake vis-à-vis the intake of other nutrients and kidney stones in healthy individuals.
Knowledge Gaps	17	A.II.08	Because of their potential to increase the risk of mineral depletion in vulnerable populations, calcium–mineral interactions should be the subject of additional studies.
Knowledge Gaps	19	A.III.02	Bone mineral mass as a function of dietary phosphorus intake should be investigated at all stages of the life cycle.
Knowledge Gaps	20	A.III.03	The practical effect of phosphate-containing food additives on trace mineral status (iron, copper, and zinc) should be evaluated.
Knowledge Gaps	27	A.IV.08	Based on the evidence of abnormal magnesium status and health outcomes [from research in Recommendation ID Code A.IV.07 (pg. 249)], intervention studies to improve magnesium status and to assess its impact on specific health outcomes would be appropriate. Possible health outcomes include hypertension, hyperlipidemia, atherosclerotic vascular disease, altered bone turnover, and osteoporosis.
Knowledge Gaps	28	A.IV.09	The toxicity of pharmacological doses of magnesium requires further investigation.

Knowledge Gaps	29	A.V.01	Research is needed to evaluate how geographical and racial variables (that reflect the mix of the Canadian and American population) affect vitamin D status at various levels of vitamin D intake throughout the lifespan.
Knowledge Gaps	30	A.V.02	Research is needed to evaluate the influence of sunscreens on vitamin D status.
Knowledge Gaps	31	A.V.03	Regarding puberty and adolescence, research is needed to evaluate the effect of various intakes of vitamin D on circulating concentrations of 25-hydroxyvitamin D [25(OH)D] and 1,25-dihydroxyvitamin D [1,25(OH)2D] during winter at a time when no vitamin D comes from sunlight exposure. During this time, the body adapts by increasing the renal metabolism of 25-hydroxyvitamin D [25(OH)D] to 1,25-dihydroxyvitamin D [1,25(OH)2D] and the efficiency of intestinal calcium absorption, thereby satisfying the increased calcium requirement by the rapidly growing skeleton.
Knowledge Gaps	32	A.V.04	It is very difficult to determine the reference values for vitamin D in healthy young adults aged 18 through 30 and 31 through 50 years in the absence of sunlight exposure because of their typically high involvement in outdoor activity and the unexplored contribution of sunlight to vitamin D stores. More studies are needed that evaluate various doses of vitamin D in young and middle-aged adults in the absence of sunlight exposure.

Knowledge Gaps	33	A.V.05	A major difficulty in determining how much vitamin D is adequate for the body's requirement is that a normal range for serum 25-hydroxyvitamin D [25(OH)D] is 25 to 137.5 nmol/liter (10 to 55 ng/ml) for all gender and life stage groups. However, there is evidence, especially in the elderly, that in order for the parathyroid hormone (PTH) to be at the optimum level, a 25-hydroxyvitamin D [25(OH)D] of 50 nmol/liter (20 ng/ml) or greater may be required. Therefore, more studies are needed to evaluate other parameters of calcium metabolism as they relate to vitamin D status including circulating concentrations of parathyroid hormone (PTH).
Knowledge Gaps	35	A.VI.01	Epidemiological studies (especially analytical studies) of the relationships among fluoride exposures from all major sources and the prevalence of dental caries and enamel fluorosis at specific life stages should continue for the purposes of detecting trends and determining the contribution of each source to the effects demonstrated.
Knowledge Gaps	36	A.VI.02	Epidemiological and basic laboratory studies should further refine our understanding of the effects of fluoride on the quality and biomechanical properties of bone and on the calcification of soft tissue.

Knowledge Gaps	37	A.VI.03	Studies are needed to define the effects of metabolic and environmental variables on the absorption, excretion, retention, and biological effects of fluoride. Such variables would include the composition of the diet (for example, calcium content), acid-base balance, and the altitude of residence.
Research Method	11	A.II.02	Calcium balance studies should be augmented with stable or radioactive tracers of calcium to estimate aspects of calcium homeostasis with changes in defined intakes (i.e., fractional absorption, bone calcium balance, and bone turnover rates).
Research Method	25	A.IV.06	Magnesium balance studies might be one indicator utilized as a marker of magnesium status. In magnesium balance studies, strict adherence to criteria suggested (IOM. 1997. Dietary Reference Intakes for Calcium, Phosphorus, Magnesium, Vitamin D, and Fluoride. Washington, DC: National Academy Press. Chapter 6—Magnesium) would improve their application to dietary recommendations.
Research Method	34	A.V.06	The development of methodologies to assess changes in body stores of vitamin D is needed to accurately assess requirements in the absence of exposure to sunlight. Such work would markedly assist in the estimation of reference values for all life stage groups.

E

Research Progress Identified by Individuals at the Workshop

For the convenience of the reader, this appendix uses information provided by workshop presenters to indicate progress related to the DRI research agenda. The list, which is derived from slides used in the workshop presentations and organized by DRI report, identifies topics that have been studied since the release of the respective DRI report and includes some current investigations. Nutrients do not appear below if no presenter noted substantial progress for them. Items in the list represent the view of the presenter; they do not represent workshop conclusions.

Calcium and Related Nutrients

Calcium

- Adults
  - Relationship of calcium intake with health outcomes—results from numerous randomized placebo-controlled trials
  - Dairy foods linked to reduced blood pressure
  - Small inverse effect of calcium on body weight—several studies
  - Effect of high calcium intake on first kidney stone and on recurrence
- Children
  - Better definition of the link between calcium intake and absorption, especially in adolescents
  - Relationships of vitamin D polymorphisms and mineral metabolism

- Early milk consumption linked to reduced fracture risk in girls and in women
- Effects of calcium supplementation—results from several intervention trials
- Racial differences in bone turnover and calcium metabolism

Vitamin D

- Responses of serum 25-hydroxyvitamin D, parathyroid hormone, and non-vertebral fracture to supplementation with vitamin D_3—a number of studies
- Vitamin D, and serum parathyroid hormone—one study
- Vitamin D and bone in adolescents— one study

Magnesium

- Magnesium depletion studies in rats
- Positive associations between magnesium intake and bone mass and negative associations with diabetes and stroke—several epidemiologic studies

Fluoride

- Relationship of elevated fluoride concentrations to bone mineral density and fractures—one study

B Vitamins and Choline

Riboflavin

- Intake data from Ireland
- Association of riboflavin intake with plasma homocysteine
- Role of riboflavin supplementation in cataract prevention

Niacin

- Intake data from Ireland
- Molecular identification of high- and low-affinity receptors for nicotinic acid
- Flushing mechanisms
- Effect of niacin on lipid and lipoprotein levels and on glycemic control in persons with diabetes and peripheral arterial disease—randomized trial

- Extended-release niacin and progression of atherosclerosis—double-blind, placebo-controlled study

Pantothenic Acid

- Pantothenic acid content of foods and/or vitamins—two studies

Choline

- Human data on male/female differences in endogenous synthesis
- Human data on functional markers— two studies
- Epidemiologic data on risk of birth defects— two studies
- Choline-betaine relationship to plasma homocysteine in humans—three studies
- Choline content of foods

Biotin

- Histone modification by biotin—one study
- Holocarboxylase synthetase deficiency and its treatment with pharmacologic doses of biotin—one study

Vitamin B_6

- Associations of vitamin B_6 and inflammation—four studies

Folate

- Associations of folic acid fortification with neural tube defects, vascular disease, cancer, cognition, others
- Association between homocysteine concentration and serum folate values
- Interactions of folate with other B vitamins and choline related to methylation status
- Mass spectrometry methods
- Depletion–repletion study demonstrating adequacy of Recommended Dietary Allowance (RDA) for folate for young women of all three methyltetrahydrofolate reductase genotypes
- Unmetabolized folic acid in serum or plasma—two studies

Vitamin B_{12}

- New methods for identifying status—in development

- Plasma homocysteine and methylmalonic acid values consistent with B_{12} values required to maintain hematological status—one study

Antioxidants

Selenium

- Twenty-five genes identified that code for selenoproteins—characterization is in progress
- Selenoprotein P as a potential biomarker for selenium status
- Effect of baseline selenium status on chemopreventive efficacy
- Selenium and Vitamin E Chemoprevention Trial (SELECT)—will provide clinical data on possible disease prevention

Vitamin E

- Much basic science progress
- Chronic disease prevention studies, especially coronary heart disease prevention in high-risk populations
- SELECT (Selenium and Vitamin E Chemoprevention Trial, a second generation trial examining protective effect of vitamin E against prostate cancer)—Is benefit limited to smokers (the only subjects in ATBC Trial)?
- Beta-carotene, carotenoids
- Dermal carotenoid concentrations as a possible new status indicator
- Chronic disease prevention trial information, with most progress in macular degeneration—Age-Related Macular Degeneration (AREDS) II will be the first large controlled trial of lutein/zeaxanthin supplementation
- Macular pigment might serve as an intermediate end point—emerging work in measurement and determinants

Micronutrients

Vitamin A

- Effect of vitamin A status on the conversion of plant carotene—one study
- The vitamin A activity of plant foods—three studies

Vitamin K

- Content in foods

Iron

- Classification of iron-loading syndromes involving hepcidin (down regulator of iron transporter)

Zinc

- Stable isotope methods in children
- Urine measurement of fractional absorption
- Fecal monitoring with zinc isotope plus the rare earth element dysprosium
- Isotope dilution method to determine endogenous fecal zinc excretion
- Partial fecal and spot urine collections
- Improved instrumentation—allows lower doses
- Zinc homeostasis and requirements for children
    - factors that affect fractional absorption of zinc and absorbed zinc
    - absorption and the "saturation response model"
    - factors influencing zinc absorption (quantities of ingested zinc and phytate)

Macronutrients and Energy

Carbohydrate

- Weight gain with added sugars from certain sources—four longitudinal studies
- Glycemic effect of the overall diet with respect to diabetes

Fatty acids

- Relationships of *n*-3 fatty acids to health
- Health effects of docosahexanenoic acid (DHA) and eicosapentaenoic acid (EPA)

Fiber

- Relationship of high dietary fiber intake to serum C-reactive protein—two studies, one from the National Health and Nutrition Examination Survey (NHANES), one longitudinal

Protein

- Linear regression of nitrogen balance data to estimate the adult requirement

Electrolytes and Water

Sodium and Potassium

- Efficacy of increased potassium intake, alone and in combination with reduced sodium intake, on preventing stroke—investigator-initiated trial proposed
- Main and interactive effects of potassium and sodium intake on bone mineral density—pilot studies underway
- Reduction in risk of cardiovascular disease events associated with sodium reduction
- Adverse effects of chronic, low-grade metabolic acidosis that results from an inadequate intake of potassium and its bicarbonate precursors—pilot studies underway
- Effects of potassium citrate and potassium chloride on blood pressure

Dietary Assessment

- Improvements in the DRIs themselves
    - Some anticipated progress on replacing Adequate Intakes (AIs) with Estimated Average Requirements (EARs) and Recommended Dietary Allowances (RDAs)

  - Some anticipated progress on better specifying factors that can alter the requirement or the Tolerable Upper Intake Level (UL) for specific individuals
- Improvements in dietary assessment methods
  - Matching of units in food composition tables to those in DRIs is nearly complete
  - Automated Multiple Pass Method for obtaining diet recalls appears to reduce underreporting
  - The combination of diet recall and propensity questionnaire may improve estimates of usual intake
  - Observing Protein and Energy Nutrition (OPEN) Study has led to better understanding of errors
  - Some progress made in quantifying intakes from dietary supplements (2 days in NHANES 2007–2008)
  - National Cancer Institute method developed for estimating the usual intake of foods, should also work for nutrients
- Better statistical methods
  - Iowa State University (ISU) method and software more available
  - Method for predicting individual usual intake in NHANES 2003–2004
- Development of tools to help professionals use DRIs correctly
  - Some progress in developing and extending software to assist users with new methods
  - Agricultural Research Service tables report proportions of the population having intakes below EARs, as applicable

Dietary Planning

- Determining usual intake distributions of specific population groups in the United States—(*What We Eat in America*)
- Relationship between foods offered and nutrient intake
  - Some insight from food folate fortification
- Food guide development and evaluation
  - New U.S. food guide
  - Canada's food guide under development using a modeling approach

- Application of DRIs for food and supplement labeling—Institute of Medicine report released in 2003, awaiting Food and Drug Administration rule
- Communication and education of nutrition professionals regarding correct uses of DRIs
    - e-learning course available for a fee
    - various journal articles
    - DRI Summary Report nearing release

F

Listing of Possible Topics for Research Identified by Individuals During the Workshop

This list, which is based on the transcript of the meeting, reflects suggestions made by presenters. It was prepared for the convenience of the reader. It should not be construed as representing recommendations or consensus statements.

Calcium and Related Nutrients

- Concentration of 25-hydroxyvitamin D—abbreviated as 25-(OH)D—needed for musculoskeletal end points/optimal circulating concentration
- Standardization of 25-(OH)D assays
- Better quantitation of the vitamin D content of foods
- Potential problem of low phosphorus intake, especially by older individuals
- Effect of the increasing use of calcium supplements on the bioavailability of phosphorous
- Effect of anabolic agents for the treatment of osteoporosis on the need for phosphorus

B Vitamins and Choline

- Cataract production as a possible end point for setting the riboflavin Estimated Average Requirement (EAR)
- Peripheral vascular disease function as an end point for niacin optimization
- Genomic effects related to possible new indicators for setting an EAR for biotin

- Possible adverse effects of pyridoxine (vitamin B_6) supplementation on the inflammatory response
- Possible adverse effects of unmetabolized folic acid in the serum
- Consideration of genetic variation and relevant parameters in determining the need for individual recommendations for B vitamin requirements.

Antioxidant Nutrients

- Selenoprotein P as a possible indicator for setting the EAR for selenium
- Health risks associated with marginal selenium intake
- Benefits of supplemental selenium as related to selenium status
- Mechanisms responsible for selenium's health effects
- The alpha-tocopherol, gamma-tocopherol, and delta-tocopherol contents of foods
- Biological activity of various vitamin E forms in humans
- The dose-dependence of carotenoid effects on health
- Effects of polymorphisms on the efficacy of antioxidant nutrients
- The role of oxidative stress in chronic disease development of biomarkers of oxidative stress
- Relationships of increased risk for oxidative stress (caused by smoking, intense physical activity, high altitude, and genetic predisposition) to requirements for antioxidant nutrients
- Predictive value of markers of oxidative stress for clinical end points
- Subgroup effects, smoking especially, which persist for antioxidant nutrients
- Should antioxidant nutrients be addressed more comprehensively for DRIs?
- Risk and benefit curves for lutein, zeaxanthin, lycopene, and selenium chemical species and modulators for possible use in setting DRIs

Micronutrients

- Roles of vitamin K in coronary artery disease and in brain function
- Human studies to examine links of neuropsychological outcome measures or other measures of cognitive function with vitamin K status

- End points related to nutrient toxicity
- Vitamin A and gene expression profiles
- Bioavailability and metabolism of menaquinones, and the roles of menaquinones in vitamin K and sphingolipid metabolism
- Classifications of iron-loading syndromes with identification of the central role of hepcidin
- The relationship between iron status and infections such as HIV and tuberculosis
- Status indices related to iron and cognition
- Food-specific bioavailability questions
- Biomarkers of zinc status, primarily genomic or proteomic, to correlate with functional outcomes such as immunity

Macronutrients

- The need, if any, for a Tolerable Upper Intake Level (UL) for functional fiber
- The lowest levels of saturated fat, trans fat and cholesterol that are consistent with a healthy diet and that may cause a low but acceptable amount of harm
- Mechanisms explaining why formerly obese persons may need 60 to 90 minutes of physical activity daily to maintain weight loss
- Behavioral, environmental, policy, and other factors that help people adhere to a physical activity and exercise strategy to help maximize their potential for maintenance of weight loss
- Consideration of differences in body composition and fat-free mass in studies related to energy
- Effects of feeding functional fibers on measurements such as blood cholesterol, C-reactive protein, microflora, stool weight
- Levels of intakes at which the onset of relevant health risks (e.g., obesity, coronary heart disease) occur

Electrolytes and Water

- For persons with kidney dysfunction, the point at which potassium intake poses a risk for harm rather than benefit
- Assessment of the protective effect of potassium-rich diets in blunting the adverse effects of sodium intake—basis for a recommended ratio of sodium intake to potassium intake

Infants and Children

- Analysis of breast milk, collected appropriately
- Nutrient intake data (especially from complementary foods) related to biomarkers that are validated in children
- Studies with stable isotopes and nanotracers to determine vitamin and mineral bioavailability, to investigate kinetics, and possibly to estimate change in pool size on different vitamin intakes
- Doubly-labeled water studies to measure energy expenditure and water turnover
- Determination of vitamin D requirements based on relationships of intake with 25-(OH)D, parathyroid hormone, bone markers, etc.

Tolerable Upper Intake Levels

- Translation of animal data to human health outcomes, which requires knowledge of the mechanisms
- Chronic studies
- Interactions of multiple nutrients and health end points
- Risk/risk models that address the risks of two different materials in a single food and differences in the risks of a single nutrient under various circumstances
- Sharper end points of adverse effects
- Dose–response analyses with larger numbers
- Depletion–repletion studies for adverse effects if feasible and ethical; otherwise, development of methods to obtain better information from cohort studies
- Validated surrogate markers of risk

Applications

- Relative importance of reducing the percentage of the population with inadequate intakes across the different nutrients
- Health and statistical considerations in selecting targets for the percent inadequate across nutrients
- Investigation of frequency questionnaires for systematic bias in intake estimates
- Determination of dietitians' methods of applying DRIs in their practices

New and Underutilized Research Techniques

- Genotyping, epigenetics, and imprinting—including the assessment of effects of single nucleotide polymorphisms (SNPs) on variability in requirements and/or ULs
- The use of first principles and discovering overlooked earlier findings
- Studying monogastric farm animals, as to find surrogate measures for dose–response studies
- Relationships of DRIs with long-term health
- Use of genetics to help predict who will benefit from a specific dietary treatment
- Use of metabolomics to distinguish individuals with a covert health problem from normal individuals and to analyze composition of food
- Assessment of methods for determining individual risk of chronic disease outcomes
- Delineation of specific genetic variants that contribute to wide interindividual variation in responses to dietary cholesterol and dietary fatty acids—considering low-density lipoprotein (LDL) cholesterol, high-density lipoprotein (HDL) cholesterol, and triglycerides.
- Identification of mechanisms whereby early nutritional experiences, such as dietary cholesterol and dietary fat intake, affect the atherosclerotic process and identification of the sensitive periods in development when this may occur.

General

- Setting DRIs for children
- Roles of genetic polymorphisms when revising DRIs
- Differential responses, based on SNPs, to classical depletion–repletion studies
- Development of a framework for establishing impacts and cutoffs for genetic variation that addresses two major points: (1) How prevalent do these polymorphisms have to be to warrant genotype specific recommendations? and (2) What is the penetrance—that is, what is the genetic contribution of variation compared to the overall variation requirement—and is that penetrance sufficient to warrant genotypic-specific results on which to base nutrient recommendations for subgroups?

- A disease prevention approach that involves targeting the molecular antecedents of disease, such as molecular antecedents for cancer
- If a nutrient has beneficial effects at doses much higher than needed for the prevention of deficiency, how should this affect the setting of EARs and RDAs?
- If a nutrient prevents an adverse outcome in one subgroup but not in another, how can this information be incorporated into a DRI process?
- Should the concept of a range of nutrient intake be reconsidered, or is there some other method to incorporate information about disease prevention (including subgroup-specific information) into the DRI process?
- Development of a standard approach for setting an AI
- Should an Adequate Intake (AI) be set for a nutrient that has no known essential functions in humans?
- Can the process of setting ULs be made more systematic—one that consistently uses a decision tree approach?
- Could risk assessment methodology be used to evaluate the lower end rather than just the upper end of nutrient risk?
- New concerns for ULs related to epigenetic effects and genetic rescue
- Can the UL concept be expanded to include a numerical value for nutrients for which an adverse effect or a toxicity has not been clearly established?
- Are separate UL values needed for different forms of a nutrient?
- Methods to apply the DRI process to chronic diseases
- The meaning of "healthy population" in relation to setting DRIs
- Setting ULs for nutrients for which there is a direct progressive relationship between intake and occurrence and/or severity of the adverse effect but for which there is no threshold
- Criteria and methods for adjusting nutrient recommendations, as for age, size
- A basis for expressing DRIs as densities or ratios
- Consumer communication research

G

Acronyms and Abbreviations

25-(OH)D	25-hydroxyvitamin D
ACE	Angiotensin converting enzyme
ADMIT	Atherosclerotic Disease Multiple Intervention Trial
AI	Adequate Intake
AMDR	Acceptable Macronutrient Distribution Range
ARBITER Trial	Arterial Biology for the Investigation for the Treatment Effects of Reducing Cholesterol
AREDS	Age-Related Macular Degeneration Study
BP	Blood pressure
CNPP	Center for Nutrition Policy and Promotion
CRIC	Chronic Renal Insufficiency Cohort
CRP	C-reactive protein
CSFII	Continuing Survey of Food Intake by Individuals
cSHMT	Cytoplasmic serine hydroxymethyltransferase
C-SIDE	Software that implements methods to estimate the usual intake distributions, available through Iowa State University
CVD	Cardiovascular disease
DBP	Diastolic blood pressure
DFE	Dietary folate equivalents
DHA	Docosahexaenoic acid
DNA	Deoxyribonucleic acid
DRI	Dietary Reference Intake

EAR	Estimated Average Requirement
EDTA	Ethylendiaminetetraacetic acid
EPA	Eicosapentaenoic acid
ERS	Economic Research Service
FAD	Flavin-adenine dinucleotide
FAO	Food and Agricultural Organization of the United Nations
FMN	Flavin mononucleotide
GI	Gastrointestinal
HDL-C	High-density lipoprotein cholesterol
HIV	Human immunodeficiency virus
IAAB	Indicator amino acid balance
IAAO	Indicator amino acid oxidation
ISU	Iowa State University
LDL	Low-density lipoprotein
MeSH	Medical Subject Heading
MTHFD1	Methyl-tetrahydrofolate dehydrogenase 1
MTHFR	Methylenetetrahydrofolate reductase
NAP	National Academies Press
NCI	National Cancer Institute
NHANES	National Health and Nutrition Examination Survey—a survey conducted periodically by the National Center for Health Statistics, Centers for Disease Control and Prevention
NHBLI	National Heart, Lung, and Blood Institute
NIH	National Institutes of Health
NYC Health Dept	New York City Health Department
OPEN	Observing Protein and Energy Nutrition Study

PEMT	Phosphatidylethanolamin-N-methyltransferase
PLCO	Prostate, Lung, Colorectal and Ovarian Cancer Cohort
PLS-DA	Partial Least Squares for Discriminant Analysis. A multivariate inverse least squares discrimination method used to classify samples
PTH	Parathyroid hormone
RAE	Retinol activity equivalents
RDA	Recommended Dietary Allowance
SBP	Systolic blood pressure
SELECT	Selenium and Vitamin E Chemoprevention Trial
SNDA	School Nutrition Dietary Assessment Studies
SNP	Single nucleotide polymorphism
SUVIMAX	Suppléments en Vitamines et Minéraux Antioydants
TEE	Total Energy Expenditure
TfR	Transferrin receptor
TNF-alpha	Tumor necrosis factor-alpha
UL	Tolerable Upper Intake Level
USDA	U.S. Department of Agriculture
WHO	World Health Organization